Living with Vitality

The Dynamic Power of Extraordinary Health

by Aaron Lloyd U. Parnell

A PZQ Press Book
PZQ Press is a division of Phyziquest Vitality Enterprizes Incorporated

Living with Vitality, The Dynamic Power of Extraordinary Health
Third Edition

ISBN: 978-0-6151-4332-3

For information address:

Phyziquest
PZQ Press Division
407 North San Mateo Drive
San Mateo, CA 94401-2417

Direct (650) 347-4565
Voicemail: 1(888) 7-Vital-7 or 1-888-784-8257
E-mail: Aaron@LivingWithVitality.com
Web Site: http://www.LivingWithVitality.com

Editor
    Alison Kaye Rhodes

Layout and Design
    Peter F. Hancik, EuroDesign

Cover Design
    Tim McGee

CONTENTS
AT A GLANCE

PART ONE
BEGINNING THE JOURNEY

CHAPTER 1

CHAPTER 9

SPIRITUAL VITALITY

PART THREE
Being There, Getting On With Life

CHAPTER 19

CHAPTER 20

How to use this book:

If you feel you are pretty-much on the complete vitality track and are just looking for the quick and simple how-to steps to make it to complete vitality:

1 Read chapter 15 first. Pay particular attention to the seven steps to complete vitality.

2 Pick an area of complete vitality to focus on, then choose one of the chapters 6-12 that correspond to your focus area.

3 Use the Resources chapter as a guide to help you accomplish your complete vitality goals.

If you would like to have an overview and understanding of the history, challenges, distinctions and opportunities that Western society has and will need as we move toward complete vitality:

1 Start reading at the foreword and be prepared to write notes and questions in the margins and spaces at the end of each chapter.

2 Be prepared to have more aliveness than you may have ever experienced before.

3 Refer to the Resources chapter to help you on your journey.

FOREWORD

The purpose of this book is to outline specifically
what being vital is and how to achieve it. You'll
understand the importance of vitality and why it is
what you've been looking for when you understand
the limits of our current health care system.

I'm happy to recommend "Living with Vitality" to anyone who wants an easily readable introduction to attaining a happy and fulfilling life. What Aaron Parnell does for the reader is to show us that we do not have to "settle" for a life that is less than exciting and satisfying. Having all aspects of our daily lives be a source of joy and to feel that we ourselves are the ones that have brought this into being is very satisfying!

Many of us unknowingly, over time, allow our lives to go on "automatic pilot" so that the quality of our lives and health become determined by others who do not have our health and complete well-being as their highest priority, such as our employers, our doctors or insurance companies, community organizations and the demands of an over-loaded time-urgent lifestyle that most adults in America must deal with. From finances and time, to holistic health care, to spiritual well-being, many of us find ourselves out of control and far away from our own values and needs in our everyday lives.

A aron Parnell helps us identify the areas in our lives which may be draining us of vitality and choice and provides us with great ideas (ones that are possible to do in the context of our busy lives) and the resources in our communities where we can find the kinds of support we need to make the changes. He also helps us recognize what our "rights" are related to directing our own health care and getting the information we are entitled to from our health care providers.

A fair measure of skepticism should be our first defense against the overwhelming pressure from the prevailing health care system to accept only one view of health and treatment so that we can make our own informed decisions about what our bodies need.

B esides this book, there's only one thing more inspiring and persuasive of the value and ease of pursuing a life rich in joy and well-being and that's meeting Aaron Parnell himself. He practices what he teaches and is easily one of the best examples of a person living with vitality that I've met.

Tedde M. Rinker, M.D.
Director, Stress Medicine Consulting
Redwood City, California, USA

We are essentially entrapped and enslaved by technology, and we've lost contact with the immediate environment. This has distanced us from maintaining a baseline level of intimacy with the things that should be most important to us—i.e., family and spiritual matters. As a result, we are in a merry-go-round that just goes faster and faster and faster. We have the false sense of security that we're going somewhere—but we're not.

This is a timely book for everyone. It trims away the fat and leaves, in bold relief, the one and only thing that's truly important and vital to life: A three-dimensional perspective on what true health is.

What you can expect from this book depends entirely on you, the reader. If you read it carefully and honestly, you will be encouraged to ask yourself questions about your only life path and, maybe, make some changes in a positive direction. Hopefully you will become a practitioner of what you've learned, as opposed to merely taking the new information and keeping it in your memory bank for memory's sake.

Health is a lot more than just the absence of disease. It ties into healthy attitudes that you have about day-to-day life, the way you handle stress, your diet and nutrition selections, proper exercise, etc. If you believe in that and implement those principles for yourself, the outcome is very simple. You will not only improve physically, spiritually, mentally, emotionally, professionally, intellectually and psychologically, but you will pass that energy on to the people around you. They will respond in a manner that either engenders a favorable response or, at least, curiosity at some level. That's usually a positive thing, but not always.

Ideally, you will attract enough positive reactions that will ultimately spread to your community and beyond, creating a healthy effect on the world. It all starts with you and how you choose to take these values and implement them in your own life. After that, the needed positive effect that it has on the outside world and your community will basically take care of itself.

James R. Lucas, M.D.
Cardiologist,
Kona, Hawaii

Let me make it perfectly clear I am absolutely appreciative of the professionals who work in our health care system. Millions of us owe our lives to this system. I greatly respect our doctors, nurses, therapists, technicians, researchers, and administrators in their ability to help people whose lives are hanging in the balance. I'm proud to live in a country that has the best health care system in the world. I am relieved to know that our experts are ready with the best technologies and services available whenever I need them.

Living with Vitality is for people looking for a sense of hope and authority about the quality of their lives in complete vitality.

Living with Vitality can have at least 12 effects on our society:

1. Parents will be instilled with hope and inspired to pass on vitality to their children as teachers and examples of what is possible in complete vitality.

2. Schools will include curriculum to teach children and young people about every aspect of their own vitality.

3. Medical schools will look for how to orient their curriculum toward the achievement of complete vitality for medical doctors themselves and their patients.

4. Medical students will choose the specialty of vitality medicine and teach complete vitality to patients as a goal for their entire lives, not just toward survival in wellness and mediocre health.

5. Commercials televised as companies channel advertising dollars into promoting the positive benefits of products that promote empowerment and complete vitality.

6. The recreational and sporting goods industries begin to promote and give financial support and scholarships for students in the vitality industries.

7. This book will add credibility to people who are already living a completely vital lifestyle.

8. This book will begin to provide a philosophical framework on which to build efficiency into a cost-effective health care system.

9. Living with Vitality opens a door for health care providers who are already in practice to go into the complete vitality business.

10. TV networks will take on the challenge of having panels of holistic care practitioners and medical physicians to answer health questions on prime time shows.

11. Complete vitality product and service businesses will thrive everywhere as people flock to them for the purchase of goods and services. There is an abundance of success-in-complete-vitality life stories that get featured on news magazines, talk shows and other media. Complete vitality lifestyle is the norm and everything else is an anomaly.

12. Healers will respond to my professional excellence challenge on a large scale and make their businesses competitive with the western medical industry.

ACKNOWLEDGMENTS

This book is dedicated to you who are on the quest for a higher level of being alive.

I feel as though I'm on a 10,000 mile expedition and I'm writing home to tell my folks what I've discovered so far. I'm still on my trip and I need to acknowledge the invaluable contribution of people I've shared this voyage with. My experiences with these people gave me the insight and awareness I express in this book. Because of them I was able to identify for myself the true distinction of what complete vitality is.

I write to you in honor of my grandmother, Suzie Mae Hickman, the Grand Matriarch of our Taylor family, who took the time and trouble to steer me in the path of responsibility and leadership.

I am grateful to my mother, Barbara Terrell, who prayed for me and provided for me along my way and continues to smile on my undertakings like an angel, truly representing God's blessings and eternal love.

I write in respect for my father, Lloyd James Parnell, who helped awaken my mind and spirit to the higher meaning of life.

Words alone, nor deeds besides, could completely acknowledge my wife and life-companion, Alicia Kaye Parnell. Thank you for believing in me and being with me on this journey. I love you. I admire you. I cherish your being.

Karl H. Croel, my father-in-law, a man whose vision has been far ahead of his time. In response to the old saying about giving your children roots and wings. You said "To heck with the roots, go for the wings." Thanks for your blessings and believing I could do it all along.

Dr. Sherman A. Nagel, my anatomy and physiology professor. You introduced me to the power of the body to restore vitality and sustain the life force. As a health evangelist, you have been a role model for me. Thank you for your caring and demanding inspiration.

In the spirit of the late Phillip Lee Reeder, my high school choir director, teacher and friend. I remember what it looks like to look for the good in other people and love them unconditionally for their gifts.

In reverent memory of Paul Derrick Larson, founder of The Summit Organization. I really see how important it is to keep my word and be true to my path. Thanks for showing me what it looks like to create a game everyone can play.

Patricia McDade, the "prophet of profit" and creator of The Entrepreneurial Edge. Thanks for inviting me to play and coaching me in the mastery game, where everyone who plays full out, wins.

Alison Kaye Rhodes, I bear special gratitude for the loving devotion you gave to this project. Your gift to my commitment to be understood has been as a translator whose specialty is making concepts easy to understand for everyone. Your talent in this process has been a wish that came true for me. I believe your contribution to the world is immeasurable. My highest wish for you is your continued success.

Special thanks to Norma Armon, Bill and Ernesta Brown, Ed and Rosalie Bullock, Deepak Chopra, M.D., Robin Rebecca Churchill, Mervyn Covey, M.D., Lois A. Flannery, Ken Dychtwald, PhD., Mark Victor Hansen, Sarah Q. Hargrave, Gregg Jackson, Charles Kokesh, Jack and Bonnie Lambton, James Ronel Lucas, M.D., Joseph T. Lucero, Market Street Church in Oakland, CA, Lloyd and Betty Parnell, Beverly Ann Parnell, Christopher Lloyd Parnell, Ulysses Gross Parnell, Faith Popcorn, Zaida Rivene, D.C., Anthony Robbins, Dr. Robert H. Schuller, John Leighton Traviss D.C., Col. Len Wallach, Andrew Weil, M.D., and Oprah Winfrey.

Special thanks to my clients at Phyziquest who have supported and believed in my work all along.

My friends, extended family, clients, staff and colleagues. Yes, this book is about the lessons I continue to learn with you during our time together. It truly matters that we had an opportunity to exchange and support each other on our respective journeys. Your contribution to my life is fondly remembered and appreciated. I continue to wish you success and prosperity.

The Purpose Of This Book Is To:

1. Introduce the concept of Complete Vitality as a greater possibility for our experience of wholeness and health.

2. Give people a realistic picture of what each of the Seven Keys to Successful Living look like.

3. Give structure to rewards, challenges and responsibilities that come with being on the quest for Complete Vitality.

INTRODUCTION

Growing up with a sickly Grandmother, I saw that a medicine cabinet full of pills didn't make you healthy. I came to the conclusion that old age made you sick and it just didn't seem right. I vowed I would make a difference by helping people live really healthy, regardless of age. That awareness was the gift of my life's work to empower people with their own vitality. That's when my quest for the secret of long and healthy life began.

The Secret Of Life = Complete Vitality

At times throughout my journey, I thought professional athletes were the only ones who knew the secrets. I also thought that special diets and exercises were the keys to health. The more I learned through my experience, research, study and work with clients, the more I realized I was looking for a way of living that went far beyond mere physical health. The secret, I discovered is COMPLETE VITALITY. To live a long, healthy, happy life, you must not only be physically vital, but also, emotionally, psychologically, intellectually, spiritually, professionally and financially.

When all these aspects of life are in balance, then you have true health - complete vitality. Being simply physically healthy isn't enough to create a happy life worth living. Wellness doesn't satisfy our quest for fulfillment in life. Complete vitality, on the other hand, opens endless possibilities of satisfying wholeness.

Making A Difference Through Massage

My quest for complete vitality began with massage. As a teenage shoe-salesman, I started massaging the feet of older people who were in chronic pain. I received so much positive feedback, it made me wonder what would happen if the entire body was massaged.

In college, I decided to major in physical therapy, which included anatomy, physiology and physics. On weekends I learned traditional Swedish Massage with Robin Rebecca Reyes and Shiatsu Massage with an introduction to Chinese Medicine under Herman Lugauer, OMD. After two and a half years I changed my major and was accepted to Life West Chiropractic College where I attended for another two and a half years.

My greatest interest at the time was massage for enhancing athletic performance. Then I read a book called Sports Massage by Jack Meagher, a former Olympic Masseur. He also used Swedish and Shiatsu massage techniques on athletes. Excited at finding a mature professional who was doing what I did, I got on the phone. My eyes lit up when Meagher complained that the Los Angeles Olympic Committee was "bothering" him to work at the '84 Summer games. "I'll go!" I said. [And] I found out how to apply.

Olympic Masseur on a Personal Mission

As an official Olympic Masseur, I gained some valuable insight about what makes world class athletes different than the rest of us. I spent that entire Summer on a personal research project studying the training secrets of the athletes. I had no intention of becoming a professional athlete, but I thought if I applied their secrets then I would win in the game of life as they did in their sports.

I identified two secrets that make athletes into champions:

1. They have a sport (activity) which allows them to synchronize their mind, body and spirit in a measurable way.

2. They have a motivating force that keeps them in the game no matter what. Winning in their activity means something to them and makes them feel whole.

I also learned their training regimes and how they stay in shape. That knowledge, coupled with my academic study of anatomy, physiology, kinesiology, biophysics and exercise science, gave me the ability to completely transform people's bodies.

Unexpected Results

I became a personal fitness coach/trainer and sports masseur. I specialized in working with "regular" people who wanted to be fit and feel good. I developed a unique system of fitness training with massage. This later evolved into a massage-workout system called, Reposturing Dynamics.

A curious phenomenon began happening with my clients. As they quickly reached their physical fitness goals, other aspects of their social, professional and personal lives began to alter.

One 30-year-old woman said, "Before, I couldn't get my husband to pay attention to me, now he thinks I'm the center of the universe! Now what do I do?" Another 40-year-old woman said, "When I was fat and dumpy, no one took me seriously. Now I'm up for a raise and a promotion and I feel great about life! What happened?" A 45-year-old man said, "The women are just coming out of the walls - I love it!"

I came to the conclusion that ones' experience of their body is at the apex of their experience of life. This was the beginning of the complete vitality concept, but still too general. There had to be more.

More Than Physical

During this time I participated in the now defunct Summit Organization, a personal and professional development company. There I earned 125 CEU credits in workshops, trainings and seminars over eight years. I gained valuable awareness and experience on the inner working of the mind and mental processing. It was fascinating to learn about how the mind makes beliefs and decisions from which we base our lives. From this course work, developed by Summit founder Paul Derrick Larson and co-founder, Alice Beth O'Connor, I created my own distinctions about quality living and the integrity of mind, body and spirit.

This later evolved into a system of mental training I use with my clients called, Para-Dyme Shift. At first it might seem odd that a fitness trainer/masseur would also coach on belief systems. [But] since my focus was on total health, it seemed very logical to incorporate the mind work with the bodywork. My client response verified that hunch.

Frustrated by my many clients who complained about dissatisfaction with their job, I devised a career development process to help them discover their LifeWork/LifePurpose. This professional aspect of life added another piece to the complete vitality puzzle.

Vision Of Vitality

My visualization and realization of what I now call, Complete Vitality would be far less than it is if it hadn't been for the most important person in my life, my wife - whom I met at The Summit Organization. A former smoker turned health fanatic, she has been rigid in making sure I walk my talk and crucial to the success of my vitality dream.

I finally put it all together: what makes a complete way of life, encompasses a fit body and balances emotions, mind and chemistry. More specifically, I identified seven aspects of life, the total, harmonious synchrony of which are the framework for an completely vital lifestyle.

Seven Keys To Complete Vitality

In this book you will learn about each key, how to understand them and what it means to be completely vital as opposed to just plain physically well. Here is a brief description of each vital key:

1. Physical:
   How your body uses energy to create and sustain life.

2. Psychological:
   How you logically process information and make decisions.

3. Emotional:
   How you feel about who you are - inner connectedness.

4. Spiritual:
   How you live based on a higher meaning in life - higher connectedness.

5. Intellectual:
   How you perceive and understand things.

6. Professional:
   How your work contributes globally to society/personally to you.

7. Financial:
   How your money adds quality to your life and value to your choices.

Vitality Coach, Posturist, and Fitness Expert

In my San Mateo, California office: Phyziquest Vitality Center, I began calling myself a Vitality Coach as well as a bodyworker.

In Vitality coaching, I lead, counsel and support people in their process of becoming Completely Vital, so they can experience more quality and harmony in every area of their lives. I help people make transitions and discover what they were born to do on this planet. With Reposturing Dynamics, I stretch and mold people's bodies so they experience complete levels of physical vitality and more.

Reposturing Yoga is the core group of stretches and excercises I assign to clients who want to experience pain-free living and enhanced sports performance.

A long with the unique mind/body technologies I've developed and teach in my work, the complete vitality lifestyle detailed in this book will take you to a new awareness of health. It is far beyond the consciousness of fat fighting, calorie counting, problem preventing, pain relieving, cancer curing and health care helping.

At present, we limit ourselves to believe that advanced technology and science is as good as health gets. Although it's fascinating and wonderful the way doctors can save lives these days, they cannot give us the sense of wholeness we're craving. We relinquish total responsibility of our health to our conventional western medical system and live unsatisfied because we don't realize the specific purposes and limits it has.

Hey! I'm Just Like You

I am not a doctor of any kind. I don't work with or study disease, disorder or dementia. I'm just a guy who wants to become more whole as I age. I want quality, dignity, and self-reliance along with my longevity. We can all create a better reality for ourselves as we consider various components and aspects of Complete Vitality. Your quest for complete vitality may be the most fulfilling journey of your life. This book is intended to be a signpost on your road map to living with vitality . Happy trails to you!

PART ONE

Beginning the Journey

The first steps on my quest for wholeness went into the front door of the first place that sounded like they were selling exactly like what I had in mind. You probably started there too.

OUR CONVENTIONAL WESTERN HEALTH CARE SYSTEM

The situation we are all in is forcing us to consider our attitudes, alternatives, and responsibility for creating a new destiny for our lives of complete vitality. The following is a glimpse of what conventional medicine is all about and how we (the consumers) can use it as it is intended.

Emergency, Illness, and Symptom Management

There are two aspects to highlight about our conventional health care system. First there is the responsive/reactive health care we see in the **emergency**, **illness**, and **symptom management** approach. When "normal" health is compromised, either by emergency, ignorance or neglect, the systems are already in place to care for us and save our lives. We're grateful our health care system exists for the countless lives it helps save.

There are ambulances ready to respond if we have a kidney failure, a stroke, a heart attack, a car accident, etc. Hospitals are pre-advised and prepared for our speedy arrival. There are tests to rule-in and rule-out the presence of illness or the nature of injury. We have drugs to produce almost any level of pain awareness or consciousness imaginable.

Research and Technology Development

There is well-financed research being done on a grand scale by dozens of research facilities and academic institutions. Researchers work diligently to produce new drugs, procedures and vaccines. Specialists replace worn-out, missing or defective body parts and can even synthesize blood. There are also new technologies for analysis and diagnosis being developed almost daily. This list could go on and on.

Our system is the best in the world at *this* kind of health care. We want our health care providers always to be able to provide us with that quality of medical expertise when we need it. We really don't want our health professionals to go out of the business of saving lives and managing disease.

The problem arises when we (as consumers) expect our doctors to personally take charge of our lives. We expect the health care insurance system to take care of the bill - no matter what the cost. A breakdown occurs when we give full responsibility for our lives to a system that was never intended to provide *that* much caretaking.

Prevention and Wellness

Until perhaps the early eighties, much of the public thought our health care system and medical technologies were assurance for quality and longevity. [But] then someone suggested that rather than *wait* for the bad stuff to happen to us, why don't we try to *prevent* medical emergencies. **Prevention** and **wellness** hit the mainstream and became buzzwords for the health conscious.

So we now have scanning tests such as mammography screening for early detection of breast pathologies. We can catch cancers long before they ever become life-threatening emergencies. Other health-risk assessment services include magnetic resonance imaging (MRI), which allows doctors to "read" the body with amazing depth and precision. We have an abounding variety of blood tests. They may suggest the presence of viruses and bacteria that could be the root of an illness we might get. There are braces, straps and supports for every movable joint to "prevent" injuries and so on . . .

In prevention and wellness programs we learn how to prevent heart attacks, strokes, stress, carpal tunnel syndrome and more. We learn how to avoid disease, illness and injury by *preventing* it - a great idea. [But] it gets very confusing, especially when we add to this what we learn about health from books, magazines, TV, news, gossip from tabloids and our well-meaning friends.

Confusion + Frustration = Apathy

We get different advice and definitions about preventive health. For example, what is a *healthier* soup? Is it better to get the *lite* soup or the *low sodium* soup? This contributes to why we get so confused, frustrated and apathetic about our own responsibility and level of involvement in our health process. In our confusion, we toss health aside and revert to our bad habits and old excuses. How many of us rolled our eyes and threw up our hands when a medical study came out saying that among other things, ketchup and hair dryers may cause cancer?

The concept of prevention is inadequate when you compare it the concept of vitality. It is like asking someone to *not* think of a banana. Invariably, with that kind of suggestion, all you can think of is a banana. In the case of prevention, all you can think of is the disease you're trying to prevent. In awareness and consciousness 101, we learn that we create what we think about.

Vitality: The Next Frontier

Prevention and wellness are not the ultimate goals for a society obsessed with youth and longevity. We really want more out of life. What we want is wholeness, peace of mind, happiness, longevity and dignity. Vitality gives us all these things and more. The problem has been that we haven't known how to achieve vitality. Most of us haven't even considered that vitality exists. So how could we know to ask for it?

We believe we can trust our health care system to give us all that. Unfortunately, conventional western medicine isn't in business to provide empowerment toward complete vitality. The system is designed to control, manage and treat diseases and injuries. It doesn't have the incentive or the experience to show people how to live a life of complete vitality. No one is taught how to look at that side of the health coin. That's generally not a part of the services the system provides. That was never the intent of conventional medicine.

Power Of The Health Care Industrial Complex

Why don't we know more about vitality? We haven't been shown or taught it. There are two sides to our current health care dilemma.

1. Ignorance Is Bliss

We, as consumers of health care, have created the system by asking it to do what it does best:

- ◆ Manage my pain and hide my symptoms. Don't confuse me with the details.

- ◆ Keep me in the game of life no matter what it costs.

- ◆ Make me believe someone else will pay the bill because I shouldn't have to.

2. Ignorance Pays

The other side of the problem is the conventional health care system itself (which we created). It has a vested interest in having us believe there is only one source for all medical technology. We are also led to believe that there is only one reliable authority for the definition and interpretation of medical problems and solutions. Essentially, we have allowed it to become a health care *monopoly*.

A great example of the monopoly in action was the debate over a bill that would decide who gets to distribute certain nutrients. Someone had the goal of making only medical doctors responsible for prescribing nutrients through pharmaceutical channels. [But] then we could only get the nutrients a doctor knew about that had been scientifically tested with irrefutable documented results.

The noteworthy thing is that medical doctors are not necessarily the most reliable sources for nutritional information. Simply put, most Western medical doctors don't "do" nutrition. There are four reasons:

1. They don't study much, if any, nutrition in medical school. They study medicine which is based on pharmacology, the study of how chemicals and pharmaceuticals interact with human physiology, not nutrition.

2. Medical doctors are extremely busy treating patients and keeping up on the latest developments in pharmacology, medical science and managed care. They generally don't have time, energy or a financial interest in prescribing nutritional products.

3. The profits made in the sale and distribution of nutritional products cannot drive the $1.3 trillion health care industry that we have right now. There isn't $1.3 trillion worth of business in making people vital - yet. [But] as soon as the demand is large enough for products and services that create complete vitality and self-reliance, then perhaps our conventional health care system will go into the vitality business.

4. Probably the most important reason MD's may not be the best source for proactive nutritional advice is that their nutrient prescriptions would be more likely to be geared toward treating and managing disease - not toward producing life-long vitality.

Remember the original purpose of conventional medicine:

◆ Manage disease

◆ Treat illness

◆ Provide a medical response to emergencies

It is unfair, at this time, to expect anything different from the system than that.

While living with this health care monopoly, we have been operating with a few major assumptions, one of which is:

We assume that the more health care costs,
the better and more efficient it is.

So we have watched the health care costs accelerate at three to five times the rate of inflation. Our health care coverage premiums have increased, while our coverage itself decreases and often vaporizes when we make a claim. For many of us, the quality of our health has diminished because we expect our health care system to do more for us than it possibly can.

With all the protection and safety our regulatory agencies have provided us, sometimes their bureaucracy works against us.

A System Out Of Hand

Many of our laws are structured with the best interests of the health care industry in mind. We are led to assume that:

If something is legal it must be OK for us; if it is not legal
or in favor with "the industry" then it is bad for us.

In this regard, the industry has become a system out of hand.

For example, there are cures and treatments that have been effective for hundreds and thousands of generations. [But] when the media positions a member of the (hundred-year-old) monopoly saying some remedy has not been "scientifically" proven, then we all automatically assume it is bad for us. If we don't quite hear "such and such is bad for you," we just assume it is okay, whatever it is.

For generations we have watched family members die of cigarette related cancer. [But] we left them alone because some "experts" in the industry said "cigarettes have not been scientifically proven to cause cancer in humans." We assumed that:

Whatever they say is good enough,
because they know what is better for us.

We have allowed them to become our mother, father, dictator and God.

Why is the system so out of hand? Until recently, for decades our cooperative health care system had been doing business in basically the same way, with relatively little public scrutiny. Nowhere are consumers (you and me) encouraged to make choices outside of what is provided for us. For example, a commercial tells us, "When you have a headache, don't take Drug A, take Drug B. It's more powerful... However, if pain persists, see your doctor... ."

If we go to three people in the same system - we're going to come up with answers that fall within a narrow perspective. [But] if we were encouraged to go anywhere we think someone might have a solution to our problem, we may increase our chances of discovering answers for ourselves that put us in charge of our healing.

This is where the limits of our current health care system are drawn. It does not produce vitality nor prevent illness. The problem is that we, the consumers, were under the assumption that our health care system could actually produce vitality for us. We were also under the assumption that "affordable" health care meant that whatever it really costs, our insurance should pay for it all. We were misled and now feel confused, disillusioned and afraid for our health and our wallets. We don't know what to do!

Who Is To Blame?

The problem is not any one person's fault. However, it is everyone's responsibility to change what doesn't work anymore. We can't point fingers at anyone in particular. It wouldn't be helpful if we could.

Not Me! It's ...

Health care professionals say it's the fault of the lawyers and insurance companies that their costs are so high. Pharmaceutical companies claim it's the regulatory agencies that force the research and development and application processes to be so expensive. Insurance companies say it's the health care providers who inflate costs and make fraudulent claims. Claims adjusters, lawyers and investigators are needed to protect insurance interests - and that costs a lot of our money.

Lawyers, who get paid no matter whose fault it is, say, "You need us because it's a tough world out there and, you'll lose your shirt if you don't have us working on your side." Some politicians campaigns are heavily funded by pharmaceutical companies, medical and law associations and insurance companies. They say we must have more coverage and more money because that's the solution to everything. "So we'll have to raise taxes, folks. It's for your own good." Even in the face of a health care mess, no one in the system has successfully been able to propose a solution that everyone else could live with.

Until recently, no one in the system suggested that we, the unaware public, take responsibility for the quality of our own health. No one said if we want to be vital and empowered, we should go to some other type of health professional who is in the business of teaching vitality. No one reminded us that since we have a market driven economy, we could just take our business down the street to health professionals who will teach and empower us to be fully accountable for our own health and wholeness.

We didn't even have a clue that we should be in charge of the quality of our own vitality. We're used to being told by advertisements that a pill or an overnight "cure" will do the trick. If that doesn't work, we're encouraged to see a doctor who will talk to us in Latin about how we need a few more tests and visits to get a closer look.

Covering "You-Know-What"

Physicians were often forced to order tests and examinations that had the primary goal of professional butt-covering. The doctor had to insure himself from the malpractice lawsuit we might bring against him because of the helplessness and subordination the system has been perpetuating. To everyone's disappointment, too much of health care has become defensive medicine. This has made many doctors and HMO's become less interested in our health problems and more interested in the number of procedures they can bill for.

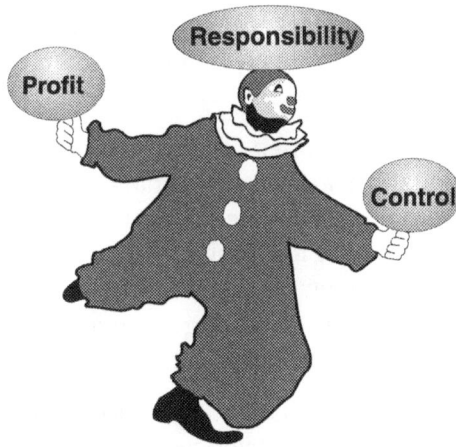

Profit, Responsibility, and Control

The complications that came with defensive medicine have only been compounded with the advent of managed care, PPO's, IPO's and capitation. What is being juggled in this confusion are profit, responsibility, and control. Depending on which group you interview, you'll find that each finds only two of the variables of primary concern.

The Real Solution

No matter who makes the profit, has the responsibility or control, it is we who must live with the solution. It is we who ultimately have the most power to create quality and vitality. It is our power as consumers to go where we want leadership. The control is still in our wallets and checkbooks and we can still choose what we want to invest our money in.

A Door To Open

We've been led to believe that the solution to the health care crisis is having more coverage for more people. Instead, the solution needs to be:

1. Set up a system that helps people create completely vital lives.

2. Encourage, train, inspire and support people to achieve self-reliance and to create vitality and wholeness for themselves.

We as consumers create the market for the services people offer. We need to start asking for empowerment and vitality in plain and simple language.

This would leave the door open for medical professionals to join forces with complementary health professionals in vitality-oriented businesses. They could empower the public through teaching. For example, if a urologist started teaching classes about how to have a healthy prostate gland forever, people would pay to come and learn. Or if a gynecologist set up a practice teaching women how to have healthy breasts, I believe women would flock to these classes.

Even more so, there would be more cooperation between the various professional communities whose science and expertise help people create complete vitality for themselves. For example, holistic health practitioners could cooperate with fitness experts, who could cooperate with hypnotherapists, and so on....

Each provider of a service could do it cost effectively by teaching a greater number of people at a lower cost per person. Lower cost for empowerment would enable more people to pay cash for what they learn. This would eliminate the cost of chasing insurance money for many health care providers.

A Window To Complete Vitality

Helping people create wholeness would be much more effective (although perhaps less profitable) than "preventing" various cancers by doing expensive screening processes or major surgery. For example, mammography screenings don't make breasts healthy, nor do they prevent the disease they're looking for.

Let's not throw the baby out with the bath water. Health screenings save countless lives and endless pain. We need screenings as part of the health care picture. They help us deal more effectively with the disease once it's recognized. [But] the question is, "How can we make our organs so vitally healthy that disease is not a reality we spend most of our resources looking for?" When vitality is our lifestyle, screenings of these kinds are necessary less often.

The great thing about pursuing vitality is that, at some point, we don't need to spend as much money with the doctors of conventional medicine because we don't get sick as severely or as often. Completely healthy people spend their money with holistic health professionals who help ensure the quality of their vitality. Empowered consumers are happy to pay for reasonably priced services that produce the results they want.

The purpose of this chapter is not to battle with the health care system. The situation we all are in is forcing us to consider our attitudes, alternatives and responsibility for creating a new destiny for our lives of complete vitality. We're simply not complete with prevention, wellness, managed care and the current health care system.

The abundant gifts of complementary medicine and holistic healing encompass the whole of life. They are waiting to be discovered by our fragmented and unsatisfied society.

Most disciplines of complementary or holistic medicine make the assumption that everything - mind, body and spirit-is related. They work through a variety of mediums to help us create wholeness and vitality. There is a broad spectrum of philosophies and approaches that contribute to one's wholeness and healthy self-reliance. The following chapter explores the truths and both the positive and the challenging aspects of complementary or holistic healing.

For further consideration see: www.AskDrWeil.com

THE COMPLEMENTARY APPROACH OF HOLISTIC MEDICINE

Many holistic ideas and practices come from ancient times. However, the idea of holistic healing is fairly new to the modern consumer's mind. This chapter is intended to help us understand how holistic healers approach their art and science.

Healers have practiced many forms of medicine since the beginning of time. Some are very limited and focused, while some are very broad and comprehensive. It is really the root from which conventional medicine stems. However, only recently has there been a resurgence in the popularity of holistic methods. Could this be because we've realized the advantages and limitations of the current conventional health care system? Has Western medicine reached the peak of its efficiency curve and started to level off?

Without discarding the lifesaving technologies of today, some people in the health and vitality fields have returned to the ancient idea that the body, mind, emotions and spirit are all interconnected. This approach to health considers the whole person and his or her life; therefore, the word "holistic" (from "whole") healing is used to describe the strategy of holistic medicine.

Here is a working definition of holistic healing:

Holistic medicine is an approach to healing that recognizes the relationship between mind, body, emotions, spirit, lifestyle and environment. Holistic medicine acknowledges that change in one area will affect healing in another.

At first, we learned to think that holistic healing is "holistic" because to some, it is considered outside the "system" of conventional medicine. However, the term "Complementary Medicine" is a more effective reference because it creates a bridge for cooperation.

The Difference Between Holistic and Conventional Western Healers

As consumers, when we go to these "Holistic", or "Complementary" healers, we often find ourselves at the windowsill of an entirely different view of life, health and our bodies. This window is the perspective of holistic healing.

A holistic healer may ask the question:

"What in the person's lifestyle, food choices or personal habits, is causing them to have the symptoms they are complaining about?"

That question is very different from the way conventional medicine approaches a person's health. Conventional medicine focuses more on the symptom that is causing the complaint; then it attempts to manage our awareness of those symptoms. Conventional medicine focuses on surface level manifestations of symptoms instead of the deeper level causes of the problem.

Holistic Headaches -vs.- Conventional Headaches

Western medicine has taught us to take a pill every time we get a headache. A holistic practitioner looks at the headache as a byproduct of what is going on in a person's life. They ask questions like, "What is going on in this person's life that is causing them to end up with a headache?" Then the holistic practitioner works on the cause of those problems through his or her own method of holistic expertise.

No matter where the healer's science comes from - whether they're a "regular" doctor or practicing some form of complementary medicine - it is the approach that makes the difference between a holistic practitioner and any other type of healer.

There are many professionals operating within our conventional system who have ventured to practice using a holistic approach to health and wellness. You will know them because they will address your condition by looking at your entire lifestyle.

> *It is the approach, not their profession that makes the practitioner holistic.*

Blind Faith Goes The Wrong Way

Don't be fooled. There are impurities to be aware of in the holistic health industry, too. It is important for the consumer to maintain responsibility for his or her health. Just because a practitioner practices a "holistic medicine" doesn't mean it's okay to have blind faith. The only person who is sure to have your best interests in mind is *you*.

Until now we have been satisfied with being seen by our doctors. We go into our doctor's office and he says, "Take two of these; they'll make you feel better." We say, "Thanks, Doc." We thought that was all we needed to take good care of ourselves. [But] now we're having the idea that there is more to feeling good than just taking a couple of pills when we feel bad.

A s consumers we are saying that we want to be involved in the process of making ourselves feel good *always* . We don't want to just feel better when we feel bad. We want to feel great and better, versus bad and then better. We want the causes to be addressed, not only the surface level symptoms. We want the problem to go away for good, not just temporary relief from the symptom.

One factor in the success of many holistic practitioners is that they teach and involve their clients and patients in the process of their own healing. However, there are two problems that holistic medicine has that prevents it from reaching the mainstream faster.

1. Teach In Simple Language

The first is that too many holistic healers still aren't teaching and empowering their clients and patients. They aren't explaining why their science works in ways that the average person can understand and easily repeat to their friends and family.

Sometimes this is due to language and cultural challenges, as with Ayurvedic medicine from India or the wealth of tribal herbal medicines from indigenous cultures on every continent.

Sometimes the practice has been professionally challenged because of unfair competition. In the case of the American Medical Association vs. the American Chiropractic Association, it was proven that the AMA engaged in a campaign to discredit and eliminate the chiropractic profession for over 40 years.

Many holistic healers have been imprisoned and had their research confiscated by government agencies. Some leave the country to avoid persecution and they take their scientific expertise with them.

Holistic *Is* Scientific

Most people are not aware that there is plenty of science behind the application and practice of almost every avenue of holistic medicine. It's just that many records from the sciences have either been lost, destroyed or were never written down.

For example, we know that the science of Chinese medicine has been in practice for over 5,000 years. Throughout that time there were millions of experiments done on the causes and effects of different modes of treatment. Many of the recorded results of those experiments are still in their original language. The Chinese medicine that is in practice today is a result of several centuries of research, practice, education and training.

With herbal medicine, many women healers have been labeled as witches throughout history and burned at the stake. Much of their knowledge died with them. Some healing practices have survived, but much of the recorded research doesn't exist anymore. The old case studies and diagrams of how the healing practices worked are the missing proof of how effective that healing art is. Midwifery is one healing art that has barely survived thanks to discrediting propaganda of organized Western medicine.

2. Operation Of Cooperation

The second problem in holistic medicine is that there is very little cooperation between the holistic professions. For example, we don't often see chiropractors openly and regularly comparing notes or trading secrets with herbalists. Nor do we hear of M.D.s regularly referring patients to acupuncturists, or naturopaths sharing findings with practitioners of Ayurvedic medicine. Because of this lack of cooperation, in recent history holistic medicine has been discredited. This separateness has left them vulnerable as businesses.

One of the greatest strengths of conventional medicine is that there is considerable cooperation among its specialists. If we have a problem when we go to the bathroom, our general practitioner knows to send us to a urologist, who may then send us to a kidney specialist.

What holistic medicine needs is more cooperation among the individual professions. For example, naturopaths should know the capacities and the limitations of their healing art. They also need to know what the other healing arts can do for a patient. That way, they can make effective referrals and support the patient's process of natural healing.

Managed Care and the Opportunity for Cooperation.

The recent advent of managed care has compelled providers from both sides of the health care spectrum to play on an increasingly more level playing field. Each party has the same interest as before: The people paying the bill to providers (HMOs, PPOs, IPOs) still want to keep as much profit and pay providers as little as possible. The service providers on both sides of the field all want to stay in the game and make as much money as they can, doing the healing work they love to do.

Only now, the rules are way different from before: for the conventional health care providers , the question used to be, "how many procedures can I bill the insurance company for?" Now it's "How few procedures can I perform to make the same money and keep this patient from coming to take up my time and resources?"

For the Holistic healers the question used to be "How can I practice my work to heal the patient and bill for it in a way that on paper it looks like a medical procedure so that insurance companies will pay me for it?" Now the issue is, "Since the insurance companies are starting to recognize the efficiency of more and more holistic procedures, how can I carve out a piece of the pie for my profession?"

Somewhere in the middle is a common language we can understand and benefit by.

As consumers we cross our fingers hoping that the full spectrum of health care services will be paid for by someone else who cares about our best interest. - FORGET IT! IT WILL NEVER HAPPEN.

The time is now for a reality check. The person who really has the power is you and me. The one truly responsible for our wholeness is you and me. No more than we would expect a life insurance company to keep us alive, we should never expect health insurance to make us or keep us healthy and vital.

Its time for everyone to make a paradigm shift toward wholeness and complete vitality. Its time for everyone to discover the feeling of wholeness and gain clarity about the power and privileges that complete vitality will give.

What The Holistic Consumer Wants From Their Health Professional

◆ Educate me about my body and how I can make myself healthy.

◆ Cooperate with other professionals I am working with.

◆ Be my partner in my quest for complete vitality.

◆ Be excellent in your work and treat me with respect.

What the health and vitality oriented consumers want is to be educated and empowered by people who are on their team. We want to spend our money and invest our trust in holistic practitioners who are cooperative with each other and their consumers. We want them to be just as competent at causing the healing of the whole person as our Western medical system is at managing disease, illness and medical emergencies.

As consumers, we are now learning that many quick fixes don't really work and some are not cost or quality effective in the long run. We are often frustrated because we are trained to go for the quick fix for all our problems. We don't even know how to think about and ask for the solutions to the problems we have.

What we do know is that we will keep looking for a better way until we find one.

When we find practitioners of complementary or conventional medicine who use a holistic approach, we will encourage him or her with our acknowledgment, our grateful business and our referrals. When this happens, holistic medicine will no longer be an holistic. It will be the mainstream.

We want to know that the doorway to the holistic practitioner in our community is:

◆ A gateway to complete vitality.

◆ A path to ageless wisdom and timeless experience.

◆ A resource for time-honored techniques and technologies.

◆ A center for applying science and research.

When general practitioners want to look up information about an area of expertise outside his or her specialty, he or she can tap into an on-line cataloging service or any medical research library. Within a few phone calls, they can have just about any information they need. That level of cooperation within the various disciplines of holistic medicine would be another blessing.

What we really want is our wholeness - yes, complete vitality. What we need from all of our healers is cooperation and alignment. A healthy and profitable future awaits the mainstream and holistic healers. As consumers, we have a vision that they reach out to each other and combine the strengths of both approaches to healing to help us achieve what we truly long for: VITALITY and WHOLENESS.

3

WELLNESS versus VITALITY

"I am the picture of health. I don't have a disease. I hardly ever get sick. I rarely get headaches. I work out fairly regularly. I eat balanced meals, most of the time. Nothing is really wrong with me. So I am a very healthy person."

This is how we commonly describe our health. Like most people, we believe that because we are well, this must be a very healthy existence.

Misguided Beliefs

Look closely at our beliefs regarding health. We say that because we are not sick, then we must be healthy. We define our health in relation to our illnesses. Instead we could be comparing our health to a higher state of complete vitality.

Our vision of health is very limited. Most of us have no idea how much better our health can be, because we do not take complete responsibility for it. We have been uninformed and misinformed about our health care for generations.

We take our health for granted until something is wrong. Then we give all our power to our Almighty Health Care System to fix us.

We believe that if we are well, that is as good as it gets.

Complete Vitality = Perfect Health

I have discovered that there is a new way of looking at our health. Included in this new belief about health, is an incredibly high standard of life that all of us can have. I call it complete vitality.

What would the world look like if everyone were in perfect health? How would we be if we were living a completely vital lifestyle? Not only would we be free from disease, pain and sickness, we would be at peace with stress. We would no longer be victims of our health care system and the medical-industrial complex. We could live and function at a high level for over a hundred years.

Is It Possible? Yes!

We would live as though we had discovered the fountain of youth, because we would have the awareness to re-create the energy we think only exists in children. It would be a world of fun and joy!

People living vital lifestyles don't have to look like way-out hippies. Living with vitality is taking control of our lives in every way. We are responsible for the happiness in our homes, the success in our careers, the peace in our minds, the love in our hearts, the health in our bodies, and the joy on our planet. Everyone can work to achieve that.

Life beyond wellness is life with complete vitality.

Here are 12 distinctions an average well person makes and how an completely vital person views the same idea.

1. "If Pain Persists . . . "

Well people go to doctors when they are really sick or broken.

Vital people go to their holistic health professionals on a regular-not necessarily frequent basis for tune-ups. They use an holistic health professional to help them achieve the goal they have in mind.

2. "An Aspirin A Day . . . "

Well people tend to focus on diseases to prevent, pains not to get or illnesses to be afraid of.

Vital people focus on keeping their bodies in sync and in peak performance condition and in some high, quality level of natural health that is acceptable to them.

3. "For Aches And Pains, Take . . . "

When well people get aches and pains, they get a prescription or over-the-counter drug like an analgesic rub, aspirin or whatever will cure their pain. According to them, the pain is the problem. A pill should take care of it, at least for awhile.

When vital people get aches and pains, they stretch, exercise, get a massage, soak in a Jacuzzi or get some rest.

4. "Starve A Fever. Feed A. . . Or Is It . . . ?"

Well people think they "catch" colds or viruses that seem to "go around." They see a doctor, take some drugs and try to feel better as soon as possible. They believe that their body is doing the wrong thing when it gets sick and has pain. So they do whatever it takes to kill the pain or cover the symptoms with medicines. They think the problem is that it's "hay fever season." Actually the problem is that their immune system is not strong enough to maintain their health in that environment.

Vital people rarely get sick or "catch" anything from anyone. If they get a sniffle, they realize it's the body's way of dealing with challenges in their lifestyle, environment, emotions or food choices. These emotional, physiological or psychological stresses have to affect the body somehow. The most common way is through a fever, a sneeze or a cough.

When this happens, the vital person goes to see a chiropractor, acupuncturist, homeopath, masseur, etc. An holistic health professional is happy to see the body releasing toxins and helps to enhance the function of the immune system through his own special techniques. Additionally, vital people may take large doses of nutrients, drink lots of water and get more than plenty of rest.

Because they do not numb themselves to the pain, they are more in touch with their bodies. They understand the natural and normal process the body has to go through to get better.

They accept the discomfort of the body healing itself because they are aware that this will bring the immune system to full strength. It will then enable them to respond more appropriately to the stresses of life.

5. "The Doctor Will See You Now."

Well people assume their doctor is "God-like" and give him or her their power. They subordinate themselves and second guess their own capacity for self-reliance in health.

Simultaneously, they have an attitude of mistrust and fear. They expect to be frustrated because they do not understand what their doctors are saying or doing. They expect to be disappointed because deep down inside they know that they are the only ones who should care enough to take responsibility for their own health. [But] they feel they don't know how.

The health care system we have right now is not designed to give us power over our lives. It is wrong for us to think it should.

Vital people assume their health professional, complementary or conventional, has an area of expertise, but with limitations. As a resource they can employ, they use them to add quality to their lives. There is an attitude of mutual respect and an expectation of trust and confidence.

6. "What Are You Covered For?"

Well people often allow their insurance carriers to manipulate them. They only get well to the extent their insurance will cover it and only in the areas their coverage allows.

Vital people consider the quality of their health first, along with the quality of their lives. Secondly, they look for the professionals who can coach, teach and empower them toward their goal. Price and method of payment are a consideration only after they have chosen their experts and are assured of the possibility of an acceptable level of success.

7. "What's Wrong With Me?"

Well people believe that pain is a problem and should be avoided at all costs.

Vital people believe that problems cause pain. They actively work and research to discover the real root causes of their problem in order to fix it in the most natural way possible.

When we're really stressed out, our natural defenses are down because of lack of sleep, unhealthy diet, negative work environment and relationship problems. This could be for any number of reasons, for example:

Picture a fort full of soldiers inside our bodies. Let's say our soldiers are living on a few hours of rest and fried foods; they don't get along with their Lieutenant Commander and their spouses are always complaining about money. They are not going to be strong enough to fight off the enemies that are constantly invading the body and will have to surrender to the "hay fever" enemy.

Why, however, are the soldiers in a vital fortress known as the strongest in the land? They get just the right amount of sleep. They eat plenty of fruits, vegetables and grains, and limit their meat intake. They drink lots of water. They are conscious about creating a positive work environment.

They are well paid. They take care of their responsibilities appropriately. They attend awareness seminars to get better informed about how to understand themselves and have great relationships. [And] they have great sex lives.

8. "An Ounce Of Prevention . . . "

Well people get checkups to see if anything is wrong with their bodies. If the doctor can't find anything wrong, they assume they are well.

Vital people get regular tune-ups to keep their bodies driving on the highway of health. They also ask questions that will empower them, such as: "Why is that?" "How is that?" or "How can I . . .?" They refuse to accept answers like "Because I said so" from any professional to whom they pay money.

9. "Doc, I've Got This Pain . . . "

Well people are limitation motivated. For example, they decide to play basketball for the first time in years. When they painfully discover that a part of their body isn't working as well as it should, they go to the doctor expecting a quick "fix."

Vital people are involvement and performance motivated. They decide they want to play basketball again for the first time in years. Then they go about finding out how they can do it sooner, better, longer, easier, faster and stronger without hurting themselves.

10. "Why Do These Things Always Happen To Me?"

Well people can't understand why things are happening to them. They are completely bewildered when they end up with a severe ulcer, for example. They are frustrated because they have to accept solutions they don't understand or trust. They give the responsibility for their health to a system that is not designed to support or empower them in vitality.

Vital people realize there are complex and direct relationships between their bodies, thoughts, actions and lifestyles. They recognize and seek things they can do to effect positive changes in their lives. They live by their own rules since they know they are ultimately responsible for the quality of their lives.

11. "We All Gotta Die Of Something."

Well people figure they have to die of something. They have a laundry list of reasons why they can't quit their most destructive habits. Secretly, they expect and fear the diagnosis of terminal illness. "Maybe then I'll do something about it," they think to themselves.

Vital people often have a vice that they balance with a set of compensatory, positive and constructive habits. They experiment with alternatives to their vice because their vice does not reflect who they think they are. They expect that as they evolve and grow, they will find a solution to their challenge.

12. "They Just Don't Make 'em Like They Used To."

Well people often refer to a time in the past or in the future when things were or might be better for them. "Back in those days . . . " they remember or "by then . . . " they hope. [And] the same old story goes on and on. They don't pay any attention to what is happening to them now. They are so wrapped up in things from the past or what they want in the future.

Vital people are very present about their interests, accomplishments and capabilities. They are aware of what is happening to them. If something bad happens to them, like they get sick, they realize how they might have contributed to this negative energy and they learn from it. If they have an excuse at all it's for why they aren't even more successful than we think they are. They rarely have regrets.

After my own experiences and observing behaviors of hundreds of people for over 10 years in my profession, the difference between being well and being vital is like night and day. You and I need to appreciate those distinctions if we ever want to have the chance for quality and dignity with longevity.

The World Health Organization does a fair job when it defines WELLNESS as:

> *"A complete physical, mental and social well being and not merely the absence of disease or infirmity."*

Here is a simplified working definition of complete VITALITY:

> *"Complete vitality is the simultaneous peak performance of your mind, body and spirit. "*

It assumes that lifestyle and personal choices contribute to improve ones quality of life.

If we want to accept the challenge of evolving toward complete vitality, we have to assume that it requires diligence and a high degree of interest. The way I thought about it was, "Hey, if I'm going to work hard and get old anyway, I might as well work hard to be vital and live a long life with quality and dignity."

How Western Medicine Thrives

Disease, illness, accidents and ignorance are a fact of life for well people.

Our model of wellness drives a multi-trillion dollar medical-industrial complex which has interests and extensions in almost everything: medical research, equipment, traditional Western medicine as a practice, hospitals, pharmaceuticals, rehabilitation, insurance, the legislature, media, the traditional structure of the corporation as God, big business' lack of concern for the environment, educational institutions and public ignorance.

The medical-industrial complex thrives on our lack of information and abandoned responsibility. This creates tremendous extra stress in our lives. In turn, the way we deal with these stresses puts our lives and our checkbooks at their mercy. The more we are disempowered, subordinate and unconscious, the more money they can make from our frustrated, overwhelmed, paranoid, stressed out and sick existence.

How Vitality Thrives

Empowerment, full responsibility and awareness are a reality for completely vital people.

The model of complete vitality drives the sports and recreation industries, personal development programs, education, holistic medicine, re-engineering of corporations, environmental consciousness, world peace, love and harmony. Its all in there.

Vital people see stress as a challenge, a learning opportunity and an experience.

They concentrate on finding ways to channel stressful energies into making a positive difference. They are participating in an evolving process of life and are not waiting around for life to happen to them.

4

THE REAL TRUTH ABOUT STRESS

Our culture has taught us that stress is bad. We believe stress is an enemy chasing us down mercilessly, aiming to shoot. We try to run away in every direction, but we can't escape the enemy's fire. We just get more stressed-out about stress.

When we are in bed with a cold, headache or body pain, we think all we need to do is eliminate the pain stress causes and we'll be safe. It's at these desperate times in our lives when we're in so much pain that we turn to the advice of TV commercials that say . . ."

When backache slows you down, just take two of these pills that will cure your pain for up to eight hours . . . " or, "Feeling irregular? This stuff works overnight, predictably every time."

Stress - The Center Of Our Health Problems

We are easily convinced to believe pills or surgery are our only escape. All our troubles will be solved and we can get back to our "normal" state of being, free from worry. [But] just in case the enemy strikes again, we're prepared because we've got our medicine cabinets stocked!

Our wellness guns are loaded with pain pills and cocked. We're ready for Stress to strike any time. We know how these stressful characters do business. [And] when they strike, we shoot them back with a round or two of drugs.

When the smoke clears, the pain is gone. We believe all our troubles are over and life in the neighborhood can get back to normal. As we go about our business, we're unaware that stress is already preparing to strike again. [And] the tradition of the stress saga continues.

We picture stress as this bad being outside ourselves with whom we have to make war to have peace. Although we win many battles with stress, we can't understand why we never win the war. It never even occurred to us to try to negotiate a peaceful settlement with stress.

The propaganda against stress has brainwashed us to believe that it's some kind of monstrous and terrible disease. Killing it with pain pills is the only way to cure ourselves.

The Big Lie

This image of stress and how we must deal with it simply is not true. Stress has gotten a bad rap for a long time and it's mostly a big lie. No bigger load of bull has ever been believed and bought.

Stress is neither a bad being outside us nor is it after us to inflict pain or damage. A world war against stress will not cure us of it and "it" is not a disease.

Here is an appropriate definition of stress:

Stress is the physical manifestation of our perceptions of life situations that affect us.

How Stress Works

What causes stress varies from person to person. We all have different perceptions of the same situation. [But] no matter what it is that causes our stress, there are four ways it manifests itself in our bodies.

◆ Physiological: When we are in a stressful situation, the chemistry in the body alters. Digestion stops. Blood chemicals change ratios and proportions. Heart and breathing rates change. The exchange of blood, air and nutrients at the cellular level slows. [And] many other things happen physiologically. We begin to die when we continually find ourselves in situations that cause us to have no relief.

For our physiological body to work vitally even under stress, we must nurture it with plenty of fresh vegetables, water, fresh air, nutrients and rest.

◆ Emotional: When we are emotionally stressed out, we become disconnected from our sense of self-worth and from the core of our values or spiritual center. Our self-esteem and our sense of self-worth are often linked to our ability to cope with the environment and situations we find ourselves in.

For example, those of us with children feel good about ourselves when we make good parental decisions about babysitters, TV programs, etc. Often, however, we are constantly just beyond the grasp of control in situations with our children and feel overrun by their strong wills. We feel out of control, less than powerful and unworthy. In these kinds of stressful situations our sense of self-worth gets crushed.

◆ Psychological: When we are stressed out, our assessment of our level of competence in a situation is compromised. Our thinking and decision-making processes are altered.

For example, we normally wake up in the morning early enough to allow us to get ready for work and eat breakfast. We function well mentally and are comfortable about making good decisions.

One day, however, our alarm doesn't go off. We wake up late for work. There is no time to shower, shave, drink coffee or dress nicely. Everyone on the freeway is driving too slow and when we finally get to work, we realize we forgot our day calendar. The decisions we make at this time are decisions we make under stress. The rest of the day is as much of a mess. If we take a closer look we might think that the rest of our lives are a disaster too. What are we to do?

◆ Physical: Our muscles tighten up when we are stressed out physically and our body loses flexibility. Muscle movement is the pump mechanism of the lymphatic system. The lymphatic system is the nuts and bolts of our immune system. If our immune system can't work efficiently, we lose energy, age faster, our internal organs work overtime and digestion slows. We lose our ability to respond to environmental changes and ward off illness and disease. Instead, we become a haven for it.

Our ability to enjoy our work and our love of life are greatly compromised when our physiological, emotional, psychological and physical abilities are not functioning with vitality.

We just looked at the four physical symptoms of stress. How our bodies deal with stress differs from person to person. Another aspect to understanding stress is how it is a result of our perceptions. We can take any of the following six points of view:

Control Without Competence

There is the example of the first time we ever gave a speech or presentation. When walking up to the front of the room, all eyes were on us. It's hard to forget that feeling of absolute control.

But we also felt sheer panic, helplessness and powerlessness. We were disconnected from our ability to present our ideas eloquently and completely. We were desperately afraid to make a mistake, stutter, talk too loud or soft, say too many "umm's" or look bad. It was very stressful. That's an example of control without competence.

Competence Without Control

The classic example of competence without control is when we are in the passenger seat of a car while someone else is driving. Our foot automatically presses the imaginary brake pedal and we give our driver hell for going too fast and barely avoiding an accident. We know we would have seen that other car, pedestrian or stop sign that our driver barely missed.

Authority Without Control

We have seen many a sovereign nation being run by a dictator or prime minister who had authority in his or her country but no control. They have a title in the nation, yet may be powerless to command authority over their military or parliament.

There are countless examples of parents who are responsible for their children's behavior, yet have little control over them.

Control Without Authority

A good example is when we get a ticket for speeding. Certainly we had the control to purposefully drive over the limit, but we did not have the authority to exceed it. When we are driving faster than the law allows, we are constantly checking our rearview mirrors for the highway patrol.

How many management decisions would we make differently if only we were in charge? How often have we sat at our desks in frustration and anger about things we'd like to change?

This causes our pulse rate to increase and we feel even a little bit tense. Digestion stops and we don't think clearly. Our body pays a heavy price in the end for experiencing control without authority.

Competence Without Confidence

We've heard it before: "You can do it! You can do it!" they said. [But] the first time we ever gave a speech in front of *that* many people was perhaps the scariest time of our lives. Well, after the tenth, and certainly after the twentieth time, it seemed to get easier. That's when we developed confidence to go along with the competence we already had in the very beginning anyway.

Limited Access To Resources And Time

You have a plan. You've considered all the angles. Your team is prepared, poised and ready to go into action. However, you lack the funding to make it happen. The project is not to be—or is it? In frustration, do we abort our plan and surrender the dream? Is there enough wood to build the house? Enough bricks to build our empire? Is there enough time to get the job done sufficiently?

In the absence of time and adequate resources, we feel anxiety, overwhelm, fear, and self-doubt. That's enough to cause major stress in all areas of our being.

Having It All

Many people have the point of view that assumes a certain degree of helplessness and incompetence in life situations. They say things like, "Oh well, things happen," "The devil made me do it" or "Life is tough."

By contrast, concerning control, competence, authority and confidence, plus ample time and resources people with complete vitality assume almost complete responsibility and dominion over the conditions in their lives. They don't become stressed out. They become stress-neutral. They make peace with stress.

They constantly ask themselves, "What did I do to create this result?" "How much of this could I directly affect through my behavior, thoughts and attitude?" "And if I don't like the results here, what did I learn so I can apply new lessons next time?" Over time and with practice, vital people gain confidence in their ability to manage fulfilling enjoyment into their lives.

How we manage the situations that cause our stress affects our vitality. Vital people have an attitude of control, acceptance and sovereignty in wholeness. Others abdicate control over their lives and delegate authority. This is not a healthy attitude. For humanity to survive, our own attitudes need to be updated to The Attitude of vitality.

In the absence of time and adequate resources, we feel anxiety overwhelm, fear, and self-doubt. That's enough to cause major stress in all areas of our being.

Here's where we make the choice to continue to let stress get the best of us or we choose to do things that will direct how stress manifests itself. In a paradigm of vitality, we know how to manage stress. We know what areas of our lives need more work because these are the areas where we feel stressed. When we are stress-neutral, we have room for a vital lifestyle.

5

A WORLD OF COMPLETE VITALITY

So what does a world look like, where everyone lives with complete vitality? What does it feel like? What language do we use to describe it? Where do we go to learn about it? How can we produce it in our own lives? How long does it take? How long does it last? How much does it cost? How much change does it require?

Complete Vitality looks like a wise master and vibrant youth combined in one person. It feels like the energy and wisdom are plugged into each other - and life seems to click. The language comes from higher consciousness. It might sound cosmic to some or spiritual or religious - really, it's whatever rings true for you. We learn it when we're ready. For some, it's a near death experience that "opens" them to the bigger picture of life. For some, it's simply a burning quest for fulfillment in life.

There are endless ways to produce complete vitality in our lives. Like a puzzle, we must begin to put the pieces together until we are whole. This book serves as a guide for how to think about putting the puzzle of complete vitality together. It takes as long as it takes. The process of putting the puzzle together is the purpose of our lives. The quest for complete vitality is lifelong. It requires as much as you're willing to put into it. It takes willingness, knowledge and energy.

Where's The Playground?

Usually, we think that vitality belongs to the youth. They're radiant, full of limitless possibilities and open-minded about life, love and harmony. When children play, they have a good time. They put their spirit into what they are doing and allow others to participate with them. They connect to a wonderful part of themselves which blossoms in that activity.

As adults, we sometimes lose that flavor of life. We either move to "Practical Island" or stay stuck in "Lala Land." The challenge is balancing work to support our livelihood and play to support our inner child. When we play as adults, we like to enjoy the feelings from our youth. [But] instead of the word "play," we use "recreation," as in literally re-creating the fun of childhood. Expressing our wishes and fantasies gives us an opportunity for fulfillment in our daily lives.

When we see a person with vitality in their forties, fifties or sixties, we are tempted to use words such as "youthful spirit" or "youthful energy" to describe them. We think that vitality is at its peak in youth.

When we do that, we limit or disregard the assets of vitality that maturity and life experiences afford. We buy into the belief that the older we get the less able we are and we don't allow ourselves to continue that youth-like experience of life.

We become saggy, depressed, hunched, stunted, toothless, senile, narrow-minded, set in our ways, dependent, feeble, ashen, wrinkled, gray, sick . . . old. At least that's been our idea of what old has to be like. No wonder everyone is afraid of getting old! Except those youthful spirit people who have taken to heart the phrase "you're only as old as you feel." The rest of us joke about this phrase because we don't quite understand the truth in it. We find it difficult to visualize complete vitality.

The One And Only Answer To Life

Because complete vitality is an evolving process, it looks different to different people. [But] we can look at examples and generalizations and lead you to the boat of pilgrims setting out to explore this new frontier. For these reasons it is impossible to give you a specific formula for how to be vital. This book doesn't have a miracle answer to life. If that's what you've been looking for, you're wasting your time. One answer to life is about as impossible to find as the Holy Grail. Life is about going through the process of learning and experiencing. Unfortunately for many of us, life doesn't just happen the way we want it to - we have to make it happen.

There are two aspects of complete vitality that we need to keep in mind.

1. Complete vitality is a new way of thinking in our society, so there are a variety of ways we can try it out.

2. Complete vitality is different for every single person. What works for me may be different from what works for you. Humans were blessed with the ability to learn right from wrong. It is our responsibility to get educated about what's available (see the Resource chapter) and trust that we're doing the right thing for ourselves. So follow highest sense of awareness and allow the journey to transform you.

15 Ways Completely Vital People Live

If you're feeling overwhelmed, here is a list of 15 ways completely vital people live life. This list will give you a good idea of what you can incorporate into your own life to become vital.

1. People With Vitality . . .

. . . Focus On Participation

Completely vital people look for things they CAN do. They invite themselves and others to join in what makes them feel fulfilled. They know that participating is a great way to get motivated, stay active and contribute.

You've heard what they say about volunteering . . . you live longer. It's true because you're participating. You're being an active member of society. You feel great because you feel needed and you feel that you are making a difference on the planet. You have a good reason to live.

2. People With Vitality . . .

. . . Focus On Complete Ability

They decide to do what it takes to be able to perform at a high-energy level. If they are overweight, they discipline themselves to lose the weight. If they're flabby, they join a fitness center. If they're stressed out, they do what it takes to relax. If they want to be better at something, they say, "Gee, how can I do this activity better, faster, sooner or more efficiently and make the results last?" (see Coaching in the Resources chapter) If they are unfulfilled, they read books like this to inspire them. If they are overwhelmed, they take control again. If they are unhealthy, they stop eating junk food and find out how to eat a healthy diet. Get the picture?

3. People With Vitality . . .

. . . Focus On Enjoyment And Fulfillment

They participate in things they like to do and work at jobs they enjoy. For their fulfillment they do things that make them feel good or that will help them complete something. They make time for their recreation and know how to have fun responsibly.

(For guidance on right livelihood and professional fulfillment, see chapter 11 or call us at 1-888-7-Vital-7 and ask us about the ParaDyme Shift program)

4. People With Vitality . . .

. . . Focus On Variety

They do different things to break up the monotony of life. Occasionally, they change their schedules. They sign up for new activities to create new challenges and expand their horizons. There is no set routine in which they plan their fun. They let their energy go with the flow and feel good about being spontaneous within reason.

5. People With Vitality . . .

. . . Focus On Healthy Sex

Healthy sex is a meditation in a divine union with another human spirit. At the hormonal level, it is a state of excitement and euphoria. At the emotional level, it is a state of peace and bliss. It brings a state of fulfillment at a personal level. In complete vitality our bodies are designed to enjoy sexual pleasure often. Desire varies from person to person, but vital people are satisfied with their own level of frequency. They know how to be free with themselves and are responsible at the same time.

(see Tantra in Resources chapter)

6. People With Vitality . . .

. . . Focus On Active Lifestyles

They involve themselves in things that will put them on the go. They are less likely to have jobs where they feel trapped. They work to achieve a fair balance between their work and their personal lives, which includes the relationships they have with themselves, their intimate partners, their families and friends. They are likely to have a variety of interactions in their social lives; for example, couples going out with other couples to parties and gatherings. They consider learning an essential part of living. They are constantly taking classes, seminars, reading books, listening to tapes and watching educational videos.

(see Personal Growth Seminars in Resources chapter)

7. People With Vitality . . .

. . . Focus On Quiet Time

It is important for people to take some time regularly for private reflection to maintain vitality. They might take a whole day, an occasional weekend and several minutes or hours each day. It is a special time just for themselves. They have no reservations or guilt about taking this time. They know they need it to center themselves and meditate. They might pray or meditate to reconnect with their spirit and the natural harmony of the universe. They might just use their private time as a break or reason to get away. It's usually a quiet time in a place that makes them feel good about the world.

(see Meditation in the Resources chapter)

8. People With Vitality . . .

. . . Focus On Meaningful Involvement

They make their lives mean something. They make a contribution to the lives of people around them. They care about their community. It is important to them to engage themselves in their community. They are often the leaders of active groups around the neighborhood and the world.

9. People With Vitality . . .

. . . Focus On Financial Self-reliance

It's not about the quantity of money or buying power they have in their lives. Money is not just paper they can get things with. They see it as a form of energy. Their purpose is to create a fair exchange of energy in the form of money (see Financial Vitality-Ch. 12), time, a meal, etc. This is how they pay their way as they go. They are less likely to be dependent on their friends, family, other people, or institutions for their sustenance because they are aware of and responsible about their finances.

10. People With Vitality . . .

. . . Focus On Open-mindedness

They are open-minded about how they get to the solutions to their problems. They don't wear blinders or get fixed on just one way of doing things. They are more inclined to take another look at a way to get an answer. They look at new ways of responding to a challenge, even if it may seem unorthodox. They are willing to experiment and discover new methods of doing things. Intuitively, they have a sense of when something is the right response to a challenge. Then they trust their decision to go with it.

11. People With Vitality . . .

. . . Focus On Responsibility

Rarely, if ever, will you find a vital person waiting for someone else to motivate them into action, ask them out or extend opportunities. They take responsibility for the quality of their lives and do something about it. They are the ones rowing out to meet their ship that's coming in. They look for and seize opportunities as they happen.

12. People With Vitality . . .

. . . Focus On Learning

They see life as an evolving process where they continually meet with challenges. Through their experience in these challenges they know there is something for them to learn. They take these learning opportunities and apply them to themselves. They ask themselves, "What am I supposed to be learning from this experience?" They believe that there is a purpose for everything that happens in life . . . good or bad. They are conscious about why particular things happen to them and seek to learn what the message might be. Upon discovering the messages in life's experiences growth happens.

13. People With Vitality . . .

. . . Focus On Trust

Because they trust themselves, they can trust others. Because they are in tune with themselves, they are aware of their limitations, talents and skills... at least on some level. They know exactly what they can do and trust that they will keep their promises. Others can rely on them. Their own confidence allows them to have appropriate expectations of themselves and others. This intuitiveness into themselves helps them keep a balance in their lives.

14. People With Vitality . . .

. . . Focus On Higher Spiritual Power

Without necessarily embracing a theology or doctrine, they acknowledge there is a power that is higher than human intelligence governing all of life. They feel connected with this power and with everything in the universe. They feel a kinship with all the living things on this planet. They have the idea that the way they live affects the entire world. They feel responsible for the world in their small way. They have reverence for how their choices affect the quality of their environment and people in other parts of the world.

(see Spiritual Vitality, Chapter 9)

15. People With Vitality . . .

. . . Focus On The Moment

They live every moment fully. They take advantage of each moment. You won't find them living in "Lala Land." They are very realistic in their approach to an ideal existence. They walk the fine line between practicality and following dreams. This forces them to stay present with each moment. If they feel the need to "check out" for a while, they consciously allow themselves to do that. They take note that right in this moment they don't feel like taking action on anything. They know this mood will soon pass and let it be okay.

Exercise The Vitality Muscles

These are some paradigms by which completely vital people live. The underlying point in all the things they do is that they are conscious about what they do at every moment. It might sound tiring, but maybe that's because we're not used to living that way. It's the same as if we ran a mile when we were really out of shape - that would be exhausting. Think of this as strengthening the mind and spirit muscles. Perseverance!

When you're ready to add more pounds to the weight machine for the mind, then you're ready to read the next seven chapters. They are very short explanations of the seven different areas of complete vitality: physical, psychological, emotional, intellectual, spiritual, professional and financial. If you can achieve complete vitality in all seven aspects of life, you will be a very powerful individual. You will be living life as described in this chapter.

PART TWO

Exploring

Touring The Seven Great Cities Of Complete Vitality

Picture complete vitality as a group of seven great cities where these miracles are common realities... no big deal. It's a land far away, but the destination is possible to reach. As you journey there, you'll have to take the initiative to study up on the culture and language of vitality. Vital people make a conscious and continuous effort to be cross-cultural and multilingual. They also might enjoy keeping a little villa or condo in as many of the cities as they can.

These chapters are designed to be your tour guides into the seven aspects of the terrain, culture and language of complete vitality.

6

PHYSICAL VITALITY

We think all there is to physical vitality is looking good and feeling fine. We are only partly right. Physical vitality gives your body the ability to use energy to create life. It also includes being responsible to environmental and physical demands.

The " Beauty Is Health" Misconception

To us, the ultimate bodies are slinky fashion models and body builder physiques. The Western world is seduced into believing that looking like this is healthy because it is beautiful to us. In the Polynesian Islands, though, skinny is less desirable and large bodies are considered beautiful. So which people live more healthfully?

Most of our ideas about fitness and health have been severely limited to appearance. A model might be gorgeous, but she also might be emaciated because she is on drugs or rarely eats. A body builder might appear to be awesome, but he might not have flexibility and therefore might have a weak immune system.

Good looks are not the goal of physical vitality. Someone who is really physically vital doesn't have to be gorgeous, but they will have a radiance and an energy that are attractive. So health is not necessarily our stereotype of beauty.

The Great City Of Physical Vitality

In the great city of Physical Vitality, health is not viewed in the above-mentioned ways. Instead, the people who live there focus on their ability to use energy to promote and sustain life force. They realize that their physical well-being is sensitive to environmental and physical demands.

Physical Vital Signs

Since we are a mammalian species, our signs of vitality represent the ability to sustain life. Some of these vital signs are:

◆ Core temperature	◆ Nervous system conductivity
◆ Brain function	◆ Pulse rate
◆ Heart rate	◆ Blood pressure
◆ Reflex responses	◆ Immune System Function
◆ Respiration rate	◆ Body temperature

People interested in traveling to the city of Physical Vitality must ask themselves: How do these signs respond to physical demands and environmental changes? What can I do to influence the function of each of these essential elements?

The laws that everyone follows in Physical Vitality are:

A) Know what the vital signs are.

B) Learn how to influence each of these to function completely in a given environment.

When you arrive there, one thing you will notice is that age and gender are not an issue. These people realize that exercise, diet choices, vitamins, herbs and drugs affect the level of their physical vitality. [And] the only qualification for living in Physical Vitality is that they must at least have some knowledge of this.

In our country, people are unaware of most of the vital signs and inappropriately hold doctors accountable for that knowledge. We also hold them accountable if their advice does not produce vitality for us. This makes us dependent, powerless, uninformed and can only make us "well", at best.

In the city of Physical Vitality, people are very powerful because they hold themselves personally responsible for their vitality. Their political slogan is, "Knowledge and choice are power."

Boost Your Immunities

Physically vital people choose to learn how to boost their immune systems. Much of what influences whether people live or die, as life-threatening diseases come and go, is the complete function of the immune system. It is essential to optimize the body's ability to get rid of its own trash. Then the body can have a better chance at removing the toxicity in food, air and water.

The essential elements of the immune system are water, oxygen, nutrients, elimination, rest and movement. Without these in place, the body's system can become heavy with toxins and die.

Move Your Booties

"Movement" is almost any type of exercise or physical activity. In the great city they do a lot of physical fitness activities to optimize their vital capacity. They know that being fit is not a goal, but a way of life. To be fit, they apply the components of fitness to what they want to be able to do.

Being physically able is a main aspect of vitality, after all. . . without your health, you have nothing.

There are eight components of fitness. Each affects the vital capacity of an individual.

◆ Flexibility   ◆ Strength

◆ Agility   ◆ Power

◆ Balance   ◆ Endurance

◆ Coordination   ◆ Stamina

Physically vital people focus on which vital signs they want to influence, Then they choose the appropriate fitness components to include in their regimes.

Do What You Enjoy

There are two things that make all the difference in exercise: enjoyment and purpose. For example, a person who loves dance might want to practice ballet or hip-hop dance. A person who wants to be strong enough to protect himself might want to learn Karate and develop all eight of the components of fitness. When we do a physical activity that we enjoy, we experience a spiritual and emotional re-creation. A spiritual, emotional and psychological bliss happens to us when we tune in to our body and ask it to do something. In a way, it is a system of synchronizing mind, body and spirit.

If your destination is Physical Vitality, here are some things to keep in mind:

BREATHE: Get oxygen into your system. Besides exercise, there are several breath therapies you can do to optimize your body's ability to use oxygen: Rebirthing, Holotrophic breath work and Yoga.

EXERCISE: Physical activity as recreation is ideal. It does not have to be a sport. You do not have to keep score. The important thing is to enjoy it enough to want to do it regularly. Forget what the experts say about going for the burn. Results come with persistence, not pain. Don't exercise to be as cool as the models on TV look like they are. You must detach your judgment of 'who you are' from your assessment of 'what you can do.'

ERGONOMICS: To avoid getting hurt, learn to do activities mechanically correct.

NUTRITIOUS FOOD: Eating 'live' foods will enhance the body's ability to process energy. Examples of 'live' foods are: fresh fruits and vegetables; natural and simple foods like whole grain breads and cereals, nuts and legumes. We mustn't forget to give our body water, also an important nutrient. It cleans our body and keeps the juices flowing. Remember, if you're thirsty, your body is dehydrated to some degree. Drink 1 ounce of water for every 2 pounds of body weight. It takes discipline, but you'll get used to it after awhile. For example, if you weigh 128 lbs. You would drink 64 ounces of water, which is two quarts. One rule of caution: Never eat when you're drinking and never drink when you're eating. Diluting your digestive juices with additional fluids may slow digestion and cause indigestion.

REST /RESPITE. The body rebuilds and heals itself during sleep, so the more rest you get, the more healing and revitalizing your body can do for you. Additionally, being peacefully away and alone to gather your thoughts is crucial to synchronizing mind, body and spirit. Also, our immune system function is at its highest during sleep. It is during our rest time that our immune system can rejuvenate itself.

Our environment and lifestyles are becoming increasingly toxic and stressful. Our immune systems may be the only survival systems we can control and depend upon.

Take care of yours.

In the end what will really matter to you is your enjoyment of life. If you're able to process lots of energy and sustain life at complete levels, you know you've arrived at the city of Physical Vitality. Life there is pumpin'! Enjoy your journey and the sights of the city. Now you've got the energy to move on to the next great metropolis of vitality.

7

PSYCHOLOGICAL VITALITY

We build our belief systems from the perception of our child mind. [And] we live by them for the rest of our lives unless we become conscious enough to want to change them to responsible, adult belief systems. When and if we do that we become mature. Yes. Psychologically vital.

Some Vital Signs of Psychological Vitality are:

◆ Healthy self-esteem

◆ Clarity of thought

◆ Positive emotional intellectual and mental energy

◆ Positive sense of self, self-knowledge, self-actualization

◆ A sense of purpose in life

◆ Quest for learning

◆ Positive state of mind

◆ Inner values match your behavior & lifestyle

◆ Emotionally present & responsive

◆ Mindfulness of choices & effects of actions

What we learn becomes what we believe. [And] very often we don't understand that what we believe connects with what we do in our lives.

We're just recently opening up to the idea that men and women who witnessed abuse or were abused as children unconsciously seek partners and create relationships that promote abuse. Why does this happen? Why is it so hard for them to get out of this pattern?

The Mind Works Like A Broken Record

For people who grew up in emotionally and physically violent families, abusive relationships are all they know about relationships. They don't know how it can be any other way. Their minds are stuck on the pattern they were impregnated with as children. Since that's the only picture that's ever been in their mind, that's what keeps replaying. As the years go by, the super glue that holds this picture in the mind gallery seems to get stronger and stronger. Taking this picture down and putting up a new one takes a lot of challenging, often painful, emotional and conscientious work.

We often trick ourselves into believing that it's less painful to stay unconscious. We would rather stay victims and believe that we're so unfortunate to have this kind of thing happening to us in our lives. Instead of finding out how life can be different and better for us, we resign ourselves to this life of misery. We allow terrible things to continue to happen to us because we think that's how life is. Why bother about anything else? The mind stays stuck like an endless recording of movies, replaying the same patterns in our lives over and over again.

Change The Program

Like a computer, imagine your "mind" is the operating system with your brain as the hardware. Your belief systems are your software programs. So if you put an abusive software program into your computer, your mind will operate it the same way it does everything else. [And] these things will happen every time you turn it on until you change the program.

If you're not into computers, imagine your brain is a crock pot. The recipes you put into the crock pot are your belief systems. So if your food is turning out too spicy or bland, change the recipe to your desired taste. In other words, if you are not happy with the way you've been living your life, change your belief systems. You've got to go to the store and get new ingredients or a different recipe for living.

It's important to point out that there is nothing wrong with the computer itself. Don't think you need to throw out the crock pot. You are not a bad person. It's the programs, recipes and beliefs you're putting in that are creating undesirable results and that need to be changed.

Who You Are Is Not What You Do

Don't confuse who you are with what you do. If you're always getting into abusive situations, don't think it's because you're a bad person and you deserve that in your life. That's a mistake.

Remember. The mind always processes information the same way. The mind doesn't care what you think or how you feel about life. Even when we learn new things, we process them through the same channels in our minds. A lot of times the new information gets filtered through the old.

[And] so we're not able to be completely objective, to be open-minded or to make a complete turnaround in a day.

The following example shows how the mind works. It's a bit extreme, but that's so you can see the point clearly.

Observation Of Something

A little girl grows up observing her mother being abused by her father, for example.

Assumption And Beliefs

She assumes that whenever men and women have conflict, there is violence because that is what she's always seen. She comes to believe that this is the way life is and that's it.

Logic

The girl knows that when a man gets angry and a woman cries, she gets emotionally abandoned or mistreated. She concludes that she must be unworthy of a different life.

Resolution/Vow/Decision

Her resolution might be, "I'm never going to make a man angry. I'll show them. I'll never get close to a man." And she'll choose relationships with no future, like affairs with unavailable men. She may choose to avoid relationships with men altogether in order to avoid violence.

Resolutions rarely work well because they're based on emotional declarations rather than logical observations. We make resolutions as children, long before our logical sense is matured. Our minds stay stuck in that mode of decision-making for life unless we deliberately update our belief systems.

It's unrealistic to think that a man and woman can have a relationship without any disagreement or conflict. There are relationships without violence - but the girl in the story doesn't understand that. So she grows up avoiding any possible areas of conflict, especially with men.

The Loophole

The loophole occurs when she chooses to stay in a relationship, no matter what the emotional cost.

Action/Behavior/Attitude

It is likely she will automatically choose a potentially abusive partner because that is what her behavior and attitude will attract. [And] she will stay in that relationship because to avoid the conflict she may become unconscious of it. In other words, she will deny the conflict's existence. Because of her background, she's already convinced that she doesn't deserve anything better. She probably thinks there is no such thing as a better relationship.

Result

Even if she ends that relationship, unless she does whatever it takes to change her beliefs about relationships, she will just go on to the next violent one until she learns a new way of relationship that works. Tangibly, her relationships are potentially violent. Emotionally, she feels afraid, bewildered, confused, frustrated, angry and hopeless about having relationships with men.

Paint A New Picture

As unconscious people, our only choices are to live by our childhood resolutions, or replicate the behavior we saw growing up, because that's all we know. If those are dismal outlooks on life, paint a new one. How? You ask. Ahhhh, you're looking for the non-existent, one and only, miraculous answer again. If life were that simple, we'd all be perfect and life would be very boring.

Nothing is a coincidence. Spirit has a plan and a reason for everything, even if we can't understand it. There are people who have had horrifying lives and yet they grow up to be great contributors to society. They are conscious about what happened to them and use the lessons they learned to help others. These are examples of people who have reached psychological vitality.

To reach the great city of psychological vitality, we must match our logic with our highest and truest values. The girl in our example can't do this because her logic about life and values about herself are contradictory and distorted. She feels conflict within herself and creates it in her life. Her beliefs about life and her concept of who she is don't match-up.

When we are in a challenging situation, we must ask ourselves, "To what degree can I affect or change this, so that I can be personally fulfilled and remain true to myself?" The girl in the story will be afraid of men and/or she will be at war with men. Part of the reason why she might be at war with men is because the way she is being treated is not consistent with what she feels she deserves.

Where The Original Programs Come From

We are born into the world with a sense of specialness. Perhaps babies are even gifted with supernatural perception. [But] we soon discover from our mothers and fathers - whom we think are God - that not all things are cute and wonderful when we do them. We discover what we can and can't do. We are disciplined. Our small minds start to believe that something must be wrong with us because we think who we are is the same as what we do. All we need to hear is, "Bad boy! Bad girl! Don't do that!" We begin to lose our special innocence. We start to put in the software programs we are being fed.

Children's minds are like sponges, absorbing everything they see and learning from it. Because they have a fresh innocence, they take in everything as if it were the ultimate truth. They don't know there is any other way. [And] from their learning experiences, they create a series of beliefs to help them sum up how life works. [But] remember, these beliefs are being created by a child's naive mind.

Our beliefs are often based on the sense of reality we had during our first few encounters with the particular situation. It doesn't matter how long ago it was or what age we were when it happened. Our first experiences with anything made imprints on our minds and we formed beliefs based on our level of maturity to perceive the situation at that time.

The Positive Programs

Not all the beliefs we make during childhood are negative ones. We might see, experience and learn, that old people are kind and gentle, because we saw our grandparents in that way. So we grow up having a lot of respect and love for our elders.

Also, our negative experiences could affect us in positive ways that are useful in our lives as adults. For example, being brought up in an abusive home might prompt the girl in our example to grow up and become a counselor for abused women and children, dedicating her life to helping people have meaningful, resourceful, loving relationships. So she identifies her life work and life purpose as a result of her traumatic childhood experiences. Because of that, she can help to make a difference in the world.

It doesn't take such traumatic experiences for us to make our belief systems. In the beginning of this book I told you a bit about my childhood with my Grandmother. The frustration I had at seeing her as always sick prompted me to become a health and fitness expert which led me to my ideas about vitality.

Get An Updated Road Map

In order to arrive at the city of Psychological Vitality, we have to turn back to the ends of our awareness and refigure our non-tasty recipes or our malfunctioning software applications. This process involves separating and re-configuring our beliefs and logic systems. Our goal is to produce emotional and tangible results that are consistent with our adult reality and the emotional and spiritual values we now choose to have. This is an evolving process. It is possible to live a life of clarity and peace of mind.

To begin the reprogramming process we must take control of our minds and say what we want of our own free will. This will is a divine power we all have available to us. We had it all along. Somehow many of us got disconnected from it and we forgot how powerful it can be.

The Universal Importance Of Being Psychologically Vital

The entire universe is counting on you to choose to create a different reality. This comes from trust and empowerment inside you to make different observations, hopes and beliefs. The world is counting on all of us to do this and rekindle a flame that will reunite our cultures, communities and families. We can do this when our free will is expressed through our emotional and spiritual inner peace.

When we do this, we will see a fulfilling and contributing way to capitalize on our life experiences. We can then make new choices based on current information and realities. In so doing, we eliminate fear, eradicate racism, stamp out sexism, reframe our phobias - and we will live in the absence of war, hatred, anger and pain.

With psychological vitality, our children can grow up in the presence of peace, the abundance of understanding and the communication of cooperation. Can you imagine such a world is possible? It is. Just open your mind and let yourself travel to these golden cities of vitality. Take the first steps. The beginning of the quest starts from within.

8

EMOTIONAL VITALITY

We think that feeling good is the goal of emotional vitality. Just like being physically fit is only a part of physical vitality, feeling good is only a part of emotional vitality. Many things can make us feel good like food, sex, money, other people, favorite activities and material things. These things, by themselves, may not lead us to the great city of Emotional Vitality.

Some Vital Signs of Emotional Vitality Are:

◆ Healthy self-esteem - how you feel about who you are

◆ Ability to recognize and express feelings and emotions

◆ Inner connectedness

◆ Living with integrity - actions consistent with values

◆ Sense of higher purpose

◆ Strong support system

◆ Feeling of wholeness, completeness

◆ Reverence for self and others

◆ Ability to acknowledge emotional sufficiency

◆ Separation between who I am & what I do

We think that if we have these "things" then we will feel whole and be happy. When we finally have them, we can't figure out why we're still so unsatisfied and lost. What we usually end up doing is filling our emotional void with things outside us that really don't have the capacity to make us emotionally vital.

Filling Up On Nothing

We continue to indulge ourselves more and more trying to feel full, but instead we become obsessive. People who are emotionally wounded and spiritually void become obsessive. The thing we are obsessed with becomes our "God," so to speak. It replaces what is missing in our lives. We try to replace what is missing with "things." What will make the difference for people with obsessions is to feed themselves emotionally and spiritually. We must realize that money, power, exercise, girlfriends, boyfriends, sex or food will not take the place of self-awareness.

Here's The Map

What is the "it" that is missing from our lives? Ourselves. That's right. What we are looking for in emotional vitality is "who we are." The only way to the great city of Emotional Vitality is to know "who we are." This is not a joke. Any other way is misleading. If we are secure in "who we are," then we will not need all the outside stimuli to try to satisfy us. We will already be whole because we are secure in "who we are" and what we want.

How do we know "who we are?" We know, if no matter what we are doing or where we are, "who we are" is never in question. We might be interacting with different people in different situations, but we are secure in what we know to be true for ourselves. Our need to have status in a group, for example, is not a big deal because we know "who we are" without status. We also know "who we are" in a close relationship, with or without our mate. We know "who we are" at our jobs, with or without our jobs. People who know "who they are," go through life with peace of mind. They're able to draw their boundaries clearly for themselves.

Drowning The Sacred Fire

It's when people are not emotionally vital that they bend their rules for themselves. If we say, "I don't like that, but because I want you to like me, I'll do it for you." What we do is sacrifice a part of ourselves. The word "sacrifice" is related to the words "sacred" and "fire." So when we sacrifice ourselves for anything, we may kill off our own sacred fire. Are you killing yourself by sacrificing who you are for your relationship, power, money or acceptance? We know if we are, depending on how connected we are to ourselves and our "higher power."

Real Emotions

If the spiritual part of us is vital, then the emotional part can be too. We're not talking about an emotional person who's up and down a lot. Typically when we call someone emotional, we mean it in a negative way. It suggests that they can't control themselves. We think of them as irrational, unpredictable, too passionate and overly expressive. Expressing how we feel in an outwardly dramatic way may not always be called for. An emotionally healthy person expresses emotions freely and truthfully based on current circumstances. One thing true about emotionally vital people is that they're not living in the past at the mercy of their emotional wounds.

Wounded Emotions

We are motivated as adults by the emotional wounds we experienced as children. The difference is that emotionally vital people actively seek to heal their emotional wounds by first taking responsibility for their own healing.

By taking active steps to cause a resolution, emotionally vital people do not hold the present hostage to their emotional past by saying, "I can't trust men because my father never kept his promises." To keep our emotional capacity from stagnating, we've got to get unstuck from our past dramas. The way to do that is to learn from them and turn them into something productive in our lives. For example, a recovering alcoholic might become a counselor. A person who grew up a sickly child may become a great healer.

If, as individuals, we continue to live in our pain, what happens is, our global society begins to deteriorate. We have allowed ourselves to become emotionally driven in the absence of our spiritual and inner connectedness. When we live in our emotional woundedness, we focus most of our energy around hiding our wound and filling our emotional void.

The Curse Is The Gift

The same thing that can destroy us is also what can make us great. We are born to receive these emotional wounds for a reason. It is a part of life and of being human. It's what makes the world go round. For example, some of us seek power because the absence of it created a wound for us. Some of us seek love, money, approval, attention, and so on for the same reasons. Where would we be if no one ever felt wounded? We wouldn't feel motivated to change the world for the better.

Nine Steps To Emotional Vitality - The Foundation

To deal with our wounds in an appropriate way we can start by:

1. Acknowledging the wound itself.

2. Recognizing the GIFTS and the CURSES of our wounds.

3. Forgiving ourselves for the way we responded to living through our wounds.

4. Forgiving whoever it was that gave us our wounds (usually it's our parents).

5. Learning the lessons and seeing the good aspects of having the wound.

6. Being thankful for the wounds.

7. Releasing the drama of the story behind the wound.

8. Vowing never to live from the negative drama of the wound-but to acknowledge the present reality of who we've become and what we've acquired and accomplished because of it.

9. Get on with the rest of your life and share the good gifts you've acquired from your life lessons with others. Make positive difference.

When we can successfully do this, then we can recognize the truth of our self-worth. Mature adults have moved through their pain and expanded their range of emotional capacities. All of us are born with some emotional capacity. [And] we all express it differently, too.

Different Expressions

An easy difference to see is between men and women. Contrary to popular belief, men are as emotional as women, they just express their emotions very differently. Often when a man feels emotional about something, he'll think about it to himself. Then his emotions will drive him to create a solution. Women, on the other hand, tend to share and exchange ideas and feelings with friends before they decide what to do.

The problem we all face is when each gender expects the other to express emotions in the same way. We need to realize that men and women aren't just different sexes. We're totally different races with different cultures and languages. No wonder there are always misunderstandings and problems. We need to approach each other as if we were foreigners. Before we go to a foreign country, we study about the country, people, language and culture we're going to visit. We read books, listen to tapes, maybe even go to a lecture to learn about these different people.

Once we're in the foreign country, we become aware of things that are and aren't allowed. We don't say, "Gee, it should be different here." We certainly don't expect to change a whole country. We just accept and respect it for how it is. In response to that differentness, we make changes in how we do things knowing that "who we are" does not change in that culture. So we let go and just enjoy it. Men and women would respect and appreciate each other more if we took this approach.

But how can we make sure we don't lose ourselves in the new culture? Remember, that culture influences, yes, but does not create our identity. Although we may have to conform a bit, it doesn't damage us emotionally because we are secure in "who we are."

One way we can be ourselves emotionally is by creating or being part of a community. A foreigner in a foreign country might look for other people who speak his language to identify with.

It is equally important for men and women to bond with others of their own gender so they can build a sense of themselves. When men meet with other men and women gather with other women, they are able to express their emotions in their own language and manners, giving each gender a chance to be completely understood. This helps them in having the experience of feeling whole and complete. When people feel complete and full within themselves, they have so much more to share in a relationship.

We can develop community with any of the groups we identify with. For example: I am a firstborn son, a healer, a teacher, an entrepreneur and a husband. I immediately identify with firstborn children. I gather with a men's group regularly and I associate with other healers professionally. I recommend that you name the top five identities you have and then find or create a way to regularly exchange ideas and experiences with groups of like identities.

The Power Of Knowing Who You Are

If we were all emotionally vital there wouldn't be the kinds of violence, conflict and misunderstandings we see, and the world would be a much nicer place. That's why it's so important for parents to raise their children to know "who they are," no matter what they are doing. If children already know "who they are" when entering school, they're less likely to yeild to peer pressure. What their friends do will be less likely to lead them astray from their own identity.

How can we teach our children to know "who they are"? The answer is easy to give, yet not so simple to do. We teach our children who they are with the way they connect themselves spiritually. Keeping in mind that all a child has is his or her imagination, he or she can identify with his or her inner self by coloring, painting, dancing, singing, talking, dreaming and playing.

Imagination is something that is divine. It expresses itself through those open windows in a child's mind. When a child is encouraged to express himself, he has to get in touch with himself in order to make that expression. That is important not to forget as we get older, too. We find the same sense of connectedness when we do these very things even as adults.

Emotional Expression

It is important for people to look for ways in which to express themselves emotionally. The earlier the better, but it's never too late. We all have it in us. We just express it in different ways. Most of us can point to a thing we like to do, used to do, or would like to do that reveals our emotional selves. We must get in touch with who we are when we enjoy doing that activity.

The kinds of questions you ask yourself are:

◆ What am I interested in?

◆ How does it make me feel?

Our interests respond to our feelings. [And] our feelings are our emotions, which are directly tied to our spirit. So we can see why working at a job we don't like is killing off the spiritually expressive part of us. [But] working at something we love is driven by our passion for it.

The same thing works in relationships, too. If we don't feed ourselves emotionally, we have nothing to share with a partner. We've got to do things we're interested in to feed ourselves spiritually. When we do this, we have a whole lot to share, emotionally, especially our emotional wholeness.

Start getting to know yourself. Ask yourself,

◆ Who am I?

◆ What is important to me?

◆ What am I interested in?

◆ What is my purpose on this planet?

For example, I am an eldest son, big brother, caring husband, honest person, mystic, pioneer, philosopher, teacher, healer and entrepreneur. Your vitality is important to me. I am interested in holistic health methods. My mission is to help restore vitality to the planet and the people living on it.

What I do to express myself emotionally and connect myself spiritually is write in my personal journal, sometimes I draw and write poetry. I sculpt wood. I write dreams, wishes and prayers too. Through my prayers and meditations, I connect myself with my "higher power" - God. I also sing a prayer song that I wrote. Mine is just an example of how one may open an avenue of emotional expression.

How Emotional Vitality Will Bring Peace On Earth

I encourage you to explore your heart for who you are in your emotional vitality. If you do (and it may take practice), you will start to discover a side of you that may begin a healing process or accelerate a mission you are already engaged in. The world will change for the better because you are becoming emotionally vital.

If people are vital in their emotional lives, then things will change. I'm putting this out in hopes that parents will add something to the way they raise their children; that we get in touch with what is spiritually connecting to us; that we feel good about expressing ourselves by including new and old hobbies. When we're all reconnected to ourselves and each other, peace will prevail.

9

SPIRITUAL VITALITY

We think that the only way to be spiritual is to be religious. When we want to feel close to a "higher power", we might say to ourselves, "I guess I have to go back to church." We think that the more we practice religious rituals, the more spiritual we will become. Although this might be so for some, a religious path may not be the only, nor the best, way to reach spiritual vitality for all people.

Some of the Vital Signs of Spiritual Vitality

- ◆ A personal connection to a higher power - Spirit
- ◆ Reverence for self and humanity
- ◆ Living with integrity with personal core values in life
- ◆ Ability to trust in Spirit
- ◆ Open in mind and heart
- ◆ Harmony, joy, peace and balance in life
- ◆ Awareness of connection of divine self with higher source
- ◆ Spiritual compatibility with friends
- ◆ Expression of Spirit in everyday choices

The Purpose Of Spirituality

Many of us are misled into thinking that the goal of spirituality is being a good ritual practicer. We lose sight of the purpose of spirituality, which is the quest for higher meaning in life. We often get sidetracked by the specifics of the traditions of our beliefs. Lighting candles on special holy days, going to church or temple, making the pilgrimage, dressing in a certain manner or praying in a specific way, are some examples of religious practices. [But] how many people follow these examples and still feel lost inside or feel disconnected from their "higher power"?

The Start Of Religious Traditions

Like being physically fit is only a part of physical vitality, being religious is only one approach to being spiritually vital. Every set of religious beliefs is a way to get to spiritual vitality. Throughout history, at the beginning of every religious tradition, we find some person or group of leaders who figured out that their way was the best for them to become spiritually connected to a "higher power." So they went about sharing that way with others.

In every culture, these historical individuals devised a way for themselves and their communities to practice religious traditions as a way to achieve spiritual atonement and enlightenment. Many of them are known as prophets. What our religions have done is institutionalize their reasons and methods for living life. These methods are different approaches to achieve the same purpose - closeness with Spirit and living life to reflect the highest and truest of all spiritual and human values.

Connecting With The World

Much of how we feel close to "Spirit" comes from our national, traditional and family upbringing. How we are raised greatly influences how connected we feel spiritually. As we are taught about the significance of what is really important in life, we learn about those things in relation to our concept of Spirit.

Among those things are:

◆ Ethnicity   ◆ Country

◆ Family   ◆ Nature

◆ Gender   ◆ Gift of life

◆ Community   ◆ Love and partnership

Just as we are given our genes, height and weight and we must manage them to achieve physical vitality, to achieve spiritual vitality, we must work with our other birthrights, such as gender, ethnicity and national origin. These are examples of issues commonly addressed in religious philosophies. This explains why some people are so passionately connected to the land they come from. The significance of certain rites of passage, such as boyhood to manhood or the ritual of a marriage ceremony, also come from these cultural birthrights.

Connecting With The Universe

The reason there is so much misunderstanding and hypocrisy in many people belonging to all religions, is that we are practicing the rituals without having a deep understanding of our own spiritual significance.

Many of us are novices in spirituality and don't realize our true connectedness with Spirit and the universe.

Where Is Spirit?

Many people who are religious think that "Spirit" is outside of us, [But] just like we are born with a part of our parents in us, the soul also has a part of Spirit within it. We have the Spirit of "Spirit" within us when we are created. There is no need to do any specific thing to try to be close to this "higher power." It's already right here inside us all. [And] that's where we'll find Spirit if we take the time to tap into that which is within us.

I want to be clear and say that we are not the same as Spirit, any more than we are the same as our parents. We are not "divine", any more than the birds, trees and the rest of creation. There is, however, something that is divine about all of creation. Our search for higher meaning is a quest that is uniquely ours as human beings.

As we stated previously, if spirituality is the search for higher meaning in life, then the meaning for our lives is inside each of us. The voice of "Spirit" speaks to us in whatever language we understand. That "voice" has to come for each and every one of us as individuals. Somehow, in our moment of greatest enlightenment and connectedness we "know" ourselves and we know "Spirit" simultaneously.

Many people feel spiritual when they walk in nature, sing a song, write in a journal, paint pictures of beautiful things, do good deeds, light a candle, pray, take a bath, read a special book, meditate, give love, fulfill their purpose in life, etc.

Spirituality is the way in which we respond to the sacred within us, based on our acknowledgment of that which is divine beyond our humanity.

It's the connectedness with living our lives according to our highest and truest values.

We strive to feel a closeness with "Him/Her/It" by being good in our behaviors, practices and traditions. Sometimes we get frustrated or misdirected in our search for that closeness. Someone else's approach may not produce the same results for us as it does for them. This is not the time to abandon our exploration of the divine.

Beginning The Search For Spirit

Instead, we must begin our search within ourselves. Ask,

◆ How does Spirit manifest in my life already?

◆ How can I open myself to letting Spirit radiate through me easier, better, stronger, more often and consistently?

◆ If Spirit were me, facing my challenges,

◆ What would I choose?

◆ How would I live my life?

◆ Where would I go?

◆ What would I do?

Those of us on the path toward spirituality have the opportunity and responsibility to investigate our practices and doctrines. We must see how they address or honor the list of things mentioned earlier.

We can begin to include some religious practices that already exist, or we can create, or incorporate something into our lives that is meaningful. Somehow in the process we will begin to find a nourishing power that will come from within. The world does not need another formalized religion. There are enough doctrines and rituals to go around for everyone to be able to find something that works for themselves. What the world needs is more people who connect to an internal wellspring of spiritual energy.

In spiritual vitality, what truly matters is that we get connected ourselves by doing whatever is meaningful to us and only us. The spirit within us doesn't care what we wear, how often, nor how intensely, we practice our rituals. The spirit within us doesn't care about the religious practices of our mates and colleagues. Nor does it care about their gender, sexual preference, race, country of origin, status, income or power.

Whatever form of spiritual growth we choose should help us evolve to be more of whom we are individually - not help us be like someone else. We all have a personal relationship with Spirit. Discovering this and owning it is all part of the process of life. It is not enough to live well. Wellness is only prevention oriented. Wellness in the spiritual sense might keep us from doing 'devilish' things, but it won't help us attain the power and connection we get when we live spiritually vital lives.

Tuning In

Being spiritually vital is like tuning our inner "radio" to pick up the frequency that Spirit transmits to us. The more spiritual we are, the more often we find through our actions that we just happened to be tuned to the frequency that Spirit is broadcasting on.

We'll begin to notice, as we become more spiritually vital, that Spirit is broadcasting on more frequencies. [And] we start trusting and respecting our spiritual radios more. We start treating other radios better because Spirit may broadcast a message to us through a station someone else listens to. This is when we discover that there is something to be learned from everyone and every situation. There are no more "coincidences." We understand that everything happens for a reason because we are aware that Spirit is governing it all.

Others treat us well because they see, by the way we live, that we tune into the channels Spirit uses to broadcast messages. We realize that although all humans are unique, we are also closely connected by this spiritual bond. We understand how we all come from the same origin.

The Business Of Spiritual Radio

Somewhere along the way, someone with a good radio decided that it would be better for everyone to buy his brand of spiritual radio. Not only that, everyone should listen to the same broadcast frequency that he heard Spirit on last week. For a "small donation" to his radio station, they can "save you." And for a larger donation, they can put you in close contact with Spirit "Himself!" I'm being slightly facetious, deliberately.

Then others came along and said, "I think the spiritual radio business is a good business." So after a few hundred generations of people in the business of making spiritual radios and guiding audiences to tune to certain frequencies, now we're confused. We don't know who is right, what is misleading, what is truth or what we should believe.

We think to tune in to Spirit, we have to buy the right radio that someone else manufactured and preset to a certain station.

WAIT! WE EACH HAVE OUR OWN RADIOS! We were born with them as part of the standard equipment of human beings.

In the city of Spiritual Vitality, everyone listens to his or her personal spiritual radio station. There is peace on all fronts - religious, personal, territorial, sexual, political and national. We do not become narrow-minded or selfish.

In fact, all our stations are owned by the same public radio producer - Spirit. Once we're all tuning in, we become a society that gives life to the planet instead of sucking life from it. It is possible for us to pass on a legacy of mutual appreciation and abundance, not separation and scarcity.

With spiritual vitality we can live long enough to enjoy the quality of what we pass on to the next generation. This is important because our children are an extension and by-product of that which lies within us.

The Message Of Love

From inside us, Spirit is requesting that we extend ourselves in mutual appreciation—call it love if you want.

By any other name, it means that we love ourselves for who we are, the way Spirit made us. It means respecting others as members of the human family. It means living lives that reflect the sacred responsibility of raising our children and caring for the Earth.

The survival of humanity is dependent on our ability to cultivate a vital spiritual relationship with each other and with the Higher Power that governs human affairs. It is time for us to acknowledge our interconnectedness. It is time for us to live with Spirit in our hearts and love in our lives.

10

INTELLECTUAL VITALITY

We often think our intelligence is based on what we know. We place so much importance on education, believing that the secret to success in this world is intelligence. [But] again, that is only partly true. That is just part of the journey toward the city of Intellectual Vitality.

Some of the Vital Signs of Intellectual Vitality Are

- ◆ Mental flexibility
- ◆ Ongoing quest for learning
- ◆ Knowledge
- ◆ Trust in intuition
- ◆ Lessons learned from Life experience
- ◆ Curiosity
- ◆ Open-mindednes
- ◆ Clarity of thought
- ◆ Ability to articulate Core values
- ◆ Creativity and imagination
- ◆ Ability to learn and reason
- ◆ Ability to make effective choices

We have been taught what to think by an out-of-date educational system whose schedule is still based on an agrarian economy and harvest schedule. That same system has even taught us how to think. They've told us how to process information and in what sequence. Now we look for everything to be understandable based on some logical system. However, what we don't learn to develop through our educational system is the knowing we have inside already.

Our educational system includes our family, churches, mosques, temples, schools, TV shows and advertising. We have educational toys, video games, mentors, tutors and other teachers.

It works to have an abundance of highly competent, caring individuals whose impact on society is essential and far-reaching. What doesn't work are the outdated assumptions we have about who is responsible for preparing our children for their future and what skills and tools we empower them to use.

Please hear me clearly. Education is, and always will be, important and essential to the development of the brain itself. Early education (even from the womb) has an influence on lifelong learning. The more knowledge you can use, the more useful you can be to yourself and to society.

How We Learn

In school, we're taught to develop our senses. We learn that we only have five of them: sight, smell, taste, touch and hearing. We've learned to be concerned with only the "right" answers, which are those we can prove consistently through calculations. With this kind of linear thinking, there's no room for the intangible reality. Our educational system has cultivated us to ignore and disregard a sixth sense, our intuition. It is that inner knowing, a level of unmistakable, unexplainable knowledge that we have. Without it, we're just as challenged as a person missing any one of the other five senses.

The Distruction Of Intelligence

As children, we were taught not to trust our own sense of what we think. It is even assumed that we can't possibly know about something that hasn't been taught to us yet. Many of us as children were continually hearing adults negate our innocent intelligence. We heard phrases like, "That doesn't make sense . . . . Do it this way." So as little beings, we started killing off our intuitive sense. We came to believe that intuition is unacceptable, unreliable or inaccurate and we stopped using it.

It's not appropriate to look for who should be at fault. Who can check? And it really doesn't matter. [But] what is appropriate right now is for us to take responsibility for how we create our intellectual vitality starting today. We must do this for ourselves and for the future of our children.

Reality Of The Twilight Zone

We've all experienced some example of an unexplainable incident. If not, we've at least seen TV programs like The Twilight Zone. Here's where things occur simultaneously and there's no logical explanation about why things can possibly happen the way they do. We can only accept it if it's weird science fiction. Or if it actually happens in our lives, we pass it off as a strange coincidence or even a miracle.

Maybe someone calls right when you're talking about them - ooh. Here's a more dramatic situation where intuition is playing on high. On the radio the other day there was a story about a boy and his father who were playing "hide and seek" in the woods. After the boy got disconnected and lost from his father, a search team was called in. The old, ill grandfather insisted that he go to help find the boy, despite all efforts by others to keep him at home. Sure enough, it was the old grandfather who found the boy. What made the grandfather know that he had to go search for his grandson? What would have happened if the grandfather hadn't gone?

Remember the story about the couple who got lost in the snow with their young baby? The father promised the mother he'd go for help and be back for them. Through the toughest weather conditions he made it and his family was "miraculously" saved. This arranging of our affairs, which is way beyond our own control, is divine in nature. People who are in touch with their intuition know, accept and trust this. The rest of us, who aren't secure about our intuition, seem to come in touch with it unconsciously during times of severe trouble.

Intuition Is Intelligence

People who live in the city of Intellectual Vitality are very tapped into their intuition. They perceive and telegraph messages on a wavelength other than the five senses. It sounds hokey to those of us who still ignore the little voices, feelings and thoughts that pass through our hearts and minds. We tend to think of these "intuitive" people as kooks and weirdos. We scoff at and discredit people who know things through their intuition. When we find out they were right, we pop ourselves on the head and think, "Oh, I should have listened to them in the first place."

Real psychics and clairvoyants are extreme examples of people who have a high level of sensitivity to things that are not manifest on the material plane. [But] really, all of us have intuition. Some of us just have it more highly developed than others.

Mastery And The Sixth Sense

So how can we develop our intuition? One way is to acknowledge the validity of those fleeting thoughts that pass through our minds and our hearts. Another way is by going through the process of mastery [see Chapter 13: Mastering Vitality].

When you go through the process of achieving mastery in something, there is a synchronizing of the mind, body, thoughts and responses. A person with mastery validates his knowledge and skill through practice, application and developing intuition. It enables him to take that mastery and apply it to all other areas of life. For example, Kung-Fu masters can tell us many insightful things about life based on their experience of applying the art of Kung-Fu. It's not because a master is experienced in all areas of life. It is that he is so experienced in one area, that he can have a sixth sense about life in other areas.

In our culture, we believe that we have to be old to reach mastery at something. We think it unsafe and weird to get in touch with our intuition. We tend to also think a person's intuitive sense has no credibility until they are old enough to have earned it.

In truth, it doesn't matter what age we are. When a child is raised in an environment that honors his intuitive spirit he can develop a sense of his spiritual and emotional self. Since there is a spiritual essence in emotional vitality, a child in touch with how he feels can easily tap into his intuition. Our intuitive sense speaks to how we feel.

Honor Your Children's Intuition

To keep children in touch with their intuition, we must encourage them to express their feelings. It might start with, "What did you draw? Why did you draw it like that?" Listen to them explain it. Teach children to be eloquent and lucid about the things they feel and perceive.

Children don't have any stuff in their heads about right and wrong or reasoning and logic. Intuition comes out in their artwork, dreams and imagination. A child's intuitive sense is cultivated by giving it an opportunity to come out. Children's intuition needs to be encouraged along with their logical abilities.

Honor Your Own Intuition

Adults have to develop intuition as well. Only we've got to sift through all the layers of judgment, morality and political correctness that were put on top of that intuitive sense. We need to give ourselves permission to go with that fleeting thought and trust it if it feels right. Sometimes our intuitive sense is stronger than any other sense we have at the time.

For example, how often have we been a customer watching a salesperson do a song and dance that looks good, even makes logical sense? However, we sense something funny about it. That is our intuition perceiving something that is out of alignment with the harmony of the universe. Our intuition is talking. It's best to go with that gut feeling and go to another store or we might regret it later.

The Spirituality Of Intelligence

Being intellectually vital is really about trusting our intuition and balancing our knowledge with reason and wisdom. It's not about how much we know, or how high our I.Q. is. It's about how resourceful we are with what knowledge we have available to us, not just the information in our heads, because intuition is not in our brains; intuition comes from God.

That's right. I said it. Spiritual vitality is a balancing factor to intellectual vitality. We must have both, or what will happen is there will be intelligence without ethics, power without compassion, and knowledge without wisdom.

In the great city of Intellectual Vitality, what drives the intellect is compassion, wisdom, ethics and intuition. The assumption is that we already have sufficient knowledge, intelligence and power. Intellectually vital people have intuition as the adhesive that holds their society together. They are also card-carrying citizens of the city of Spiritual Vitality where they have friends and relatives. Here is where science and spirit can raise their children and build a peaceful future for generations to come.

Intellectualizing The Educational System

If we were to create an educational system based on intellectual vitality, we could revolutionize the world in our homes, communities, holy places and school systems - district by district. Racism and hatred would go away. We would see our sameness and oneness with all humankind. [And] the world would be whole.

11

PROFESSIONAL VITALITY

We think that having a good job with a nice company that pays well should be satisfying professionally. We join in the rat race to pursue all the things we want for ourselves and our families. [But] for some reason, we get burned out. The life gets sucked out of us and we can't quite put a finger on why we aren't personally fulfilled.

Some of the Vital Signs of Professional Vitality

◆ Ability to experience Passion

◆ Ability to make a meaningful Contribution

◆ Sense of purpose & accomplishment

◆ Ability to experience Joy

◆ Opportunity for personal/professional growth

◆ Feeling a sense of community & belonging

◆ Sufficient acknowledgment & compensation

◆ Being challenged to expand & test self

◆ Power, choice & freedom to control the outcome

◆ Congruency with personal ideals & core values

Why The Rat Race Is Unfulfilling

We find ourselves lost in a job when we don't know what our career is supposed to be. Or we're attracted to a kind of work, but down the road we somehow don't feel great about it anymore. What happened? We lost track of our purpose for doing that kind of living. When we don't know why we're living, everything we do feels meaningless and empty.

Our Purpose For Living

The bright side is that we were all born for a reason. Our lives do have a purpose. There is a special way for each person to make a contribution to the planet and feel fulfilled at the same time. Discovering our life-work is the key to making a life worth living.

We know we've arrived at the great city of Professional Vitality when our work provides something meaningful to us personally. The meaning goes far beyond a job well done. Our work makes us happy. It gives us a purpose for living. The work we do is fulfilling because we make a difference on the planet and that makes us feel good about ourselves. When we find the deeper meaning for ourselves in our work, it's no longer a drain on our lives, but a motivating force. Our work gives us energy and life.

Do A Job Or Have A Career

Unfortunately, many people waste their lives working at jobs that aren't meaningful to them. They go in day after day, earn their money and go home. Something is missing in their lives and they're very frustrated about it. Someone once said, "A job is something you do with your day. A career is something you do with your life." That is absolutely true. Let's go further and say that you are Professionally Vital when your work gives you life.

The meaningfulness of work is the driving force in the City of Professional Vitality. There are two reasons work is life-giving:

◆ It provides energy (money) to buy things that have value, like comfort, security, buying power, etc.

◆ It enhances the quality of living on the planet for ourselves, our family, our community, our country and the world. The citizens here have the ability to satisfy both sets of needs and desires through their work.

Knowing Your Life-Work

What is it that drives our personal and professional needs? It usually comes from our early life experiences. In these early life experiences, we felt that something was missing from our lives and from the world. We said to ourselves, "Gee, life would be better if . . ." Hence, we made decisions that led us in certain directions in life. Somehow, we get drawn to work that responds to those missing elements for us. It becomes a driving force that leads us to our reason for living. We then turn that into our life-work.

For example, during my early childhood experiences (see introduction), I concluded from observing my Grandmother, that when people are old, they're sick. [And] when they get sick, they lose their independence and become a burden. What I saw missing was self-reliance and soundness of body. I decided that I was not going to get old and be sick. It was such a powerful emotion in me that I decided to make sure vitality and self-reliance would be a possibility for everyone else on the planet, too. Thus, I'm living my life-work as a vitality expert.

Another person may have experienced a devastating divorce in their family and decided to be a marriage counselor. Someone else may have grown up in a very poor family and so they decided to become a successful investor. Perhaps someone had a really influential fifth grade teacher and chose to become a teacher also. From the positive or the negative experiences we have, something clicks for us and it becomes our life-work.

From Mastery to Fulfillment

When we connect with our childhood vows, we can use the passion from that experience to help us become a master in the area where we were wounded. We heal our own wound through our life-work. In so doing, we create a healing for the planet. Some discover their life-work late in life and some never do at all. In this age of opportunity for self-determination and self-actualization, it is more possible than ever to realize your life-work.

What doesn't work for us anymore is our tendency to live as though we are incapable of actively and personally healing our wounds. The future of our society is greatly threatened by our hope that others will take care of us.

An example of this is giving our authorities responsibility, while at the same time blaming them for our condition in life.

When we're not aware of what our life-work should be, then we can't be Professionally Vital. When we work at a job that does not fulfill us personally, we're not happy with our lives. This work will at the very least shorten our lives and at the very worst, kill us.

We must ask ourselves:

- ◆ To what degree does my work create life for me?

- ◆ How do my life choices reflect the work I'm doing for the planet?

If you don't have a clue, then save a lot of time and hassle and go to someone who is a professional in lifestyle engineering. This person can be a coach, career counselor, a consultant, or perhaps even a job placement agency. (See Life-Work questions at the end of this chapter.)

In discovering our life-work, it's helpful to ask ourselves, "What difference would I make on the planet if money were no object for me?" People who are very happy, successful and wealthy, usually aren't doing their work just for the money. There is a force inside them that is driving them in the kind of work they're doing. They know their life-work and they are Professionally Vital in their careers.

Identifying our life-work will accomplish five things:

1. It will give us clarity about what work we are supposed to do that is both personally rewarding *and* makes a contribution to the planet.

2. Give us a step-by-step outline leading us from where we are now to the point where we can be fulfilled through what we do professionally.

3. Give us a view of the big picture about why we're on the planet.

4. Give us a realistic appreciation of how much work there is to do for us and others who have the same life-work.

5. Help us see the limitations we have so that we can appropriately work with others who have different skills.

Finding Our Life-Work

Finding our life-work comes from a combination of our early life experiences and our qualities, talents, skills, gifts and interests. We must consider how we are particularly qualified to do something meaningful on the planet. When we have an idea about that, we can move toward what we're here to accomplish. The more we live toward that goal, the more Professionally Vital we are capable of being.

The people in the city of Professional Vitality are connected to their life-work. We can all get there by becoming engaged in our own life-work. That is when we will experience fulfillment and satisfaction. We need to go beyond the mentality of "doing a job for the money." When we journey to Professional Vitality, we will be able to appreciate work for life and life for meaning. (See Life-Work and Life-Purpose worksheets at the end of the chapter.)

A "life-work" is a work we engage ourselves in that has meaning for us personally and creates opportunity for others on a global scale. One hallmark of a life-work, is the opportunities that open to create the possibilities for others to be just as fulfilled and make as valuable a contribution to the planet as we make.

The Difference A Purpose Can Make

The communities in Professional Vitality are life-giving units of love and support. Providing a service is a labor of love. Prosperity is driven by caring and spiritual connectedness. The businesses operate with honesty and integrity because that is the only way to sustain the work of life. They manufacture products that solve human problems. They give life to a dying planet. They give resolution to a humanity that needs to learn to live with each other as one and the same, while appreciating the differences. Even the politics are inspired by performance, cooperation and service.

If every individual was living in this place, there would be full employment and sufficient prosperity world-wide. Our children would grow up and find a place for themselves in a world of cooperation and mutual empowerment. Abundance and creativity would lead us to imagine and generate a life worth living through work worth doing.

Identifying My Life-Purpose

Instructions:

Complete these sentences as quickly and 'off-the-top-of-your-head' as you can.

There are no 'right' answers, only your answers. It's okay if you have difficulty coming up with a response right away. Then use the key to interpret some of your replies.

1)   In school, I was the one who _____.

2)   In my family, I was the one who _____.

3)   In groups, I seem to be the one who _____.

4)   I always loved to _____, even when I was young.

5)   _____ has always been easy for me, natural to me.

6)   At the jobs I enjoyed the most, my duties were: _____.

7)   When I was a kid, I wanted to be/do _____ when I grew up

Because _____.

8)   If I could design my own job, and money was no object, I would

_____.

9)   No matter what, I seem to get the most personal enjoyment and satisfaction when I'm either _____, _____ or

_____.

10) Based on the simple, patterns in my responses, I think my LIFE PURPOSE(S) might be _____, _____ and

_____.

11) The unique style and qualities I bring to my LIFE PURPOSE are:

_____.

12) In exchange for my gifts, what I really want for myself is:

_____.

Life-Purpose Key

1-3) Your personality reflected by how you interact (or not) with others.

4-6) Your gifts and natural abilities.

7) Whatever you wished or dreamed of, it was because being or doing that would get you something. That important 'something' is the carrot that inspires you to do what you do best.

8-9) This is your opportunity to allow the song in your heart to be sung by you. It's what you do when you have the chance to be you. It's you in your truest expression.

10) Look at your responses to #s 1-9, then write down any themes which seem to show up repeatedly in the blanks.

11) What makes the way you do it different from anybody else. These are your talents, skills and other natural abilities at work and play.

12) These are your secret hopes, dreams and wishes. After all is said and done, having these things will make life worth living and working for.

Identifying Life-Work

Instructions:

Complete these sentences as quickly and 'off-the-top-of-your-head' as you can.

There are no 'right' answers, only your answers. It's okay if you have difficulty coming up with a response right away. Then use the key to interpret some of your replies.

1) When I was a child, _____ was always easy for me, even when no one else could do it or figure it out.

2) What really upsets me when I watch, read, hear about what is going on in the world is _____.

3) When I was a child, I vowed that when I grew up I was going to

_____.

4) Even when they said it was tough or impossible, I succeeded because _____.

5) What really inspires me is when I watch, hear, or read stories in which _____.

6) I think my Life's Work is _____.

7) The part of me that I will be healing is _____.

8) Based on my character traits (from my Life-Purpose #10-11), as far as I can tell, my role within the Life-Work I have chosen is _____.

9) The difference my Life-Work will make on the planet is

_____.

Life-Work Key

1) This is your 'gift'-a special gift given only to you. Using it well may take time, talent, and training. However, for you, it usually requires less of each than for others.

2) Your 'motivating force' in life. Few things in life bother you more than this issue.

3) Your 'solution.' It's the thing that was missing when you received

 your "wound". It also seems to be the thing that is missing behind
 your driving force in life.

4) Your 'success system'. It's the ace in your sleeve when the going

 gets rough or when things look impossible.

5) This is you at your highest, fullest self-expression.

6) (Time for a gut-feeling guess) Sometimes you know it by this point.

7) This is the story of your 'wound'.

8) The 'role you are uniquely qualified to play' within your life-work.

9) What will happen to the world when you are successful in your life-work.

These are brief versions of the questionnaires used by certified Life-Purpose/Life-Work Consultants affiliated with Phyziquest Vitality Sciences Institute.

For more information, call the Institute @ 1-888- 7Vitality or 1-888-784-8254.

12

FINANCIAL VITALITY

We believe that having "enough" money is the answer to all our problems. However, when we finally have "enough" money, we discover that it's not the answer we were looking for. When we have lots of money, we do not become problem-less, we just wind up with different challenges.

Some of the Vital Signs of Financial Vitality Are

◆ Quality of living

◆ Choices available

◆ Value of choices related to personal ideals

◆ Control over lifestyle & time

◆ Awareness of relationship of finances to lifestyle choices

◆ Involvement in the choice-making of financial/lifestyle decisions

The Key To Financial Vitality

Financial Vitality is the ability to use money to promote and sustain value, quality and choice in life. The key to Financial Vitality is using our money in such a way that the universe will support us in having more enjoyment in our lives.

In Physical Vitality, we learned that the more physically fit we are, the more we are able to enjoy life. So the more financially fit we are, the more we are able to enjoy living. It's not about necessarily having a ton of money; it's how we use what we have to bring quality to living.

Viability is a term derived from VITAL and ABLE. How able are we at living a financially, economically vital life? However we answer this question regarding our financial situation reflects how much or how little money we have in our life. How much life are we able to produce with our money and how much money are we able to produce with our life?

In the city of Financial Vitality, people have a balanced management of three things in life: QUALITY, VALUE and CHOICE.

◆ QUALITY: When we know what's important to us, then we can concentrate on that and bring quality to it. Money doesn't create quality. We create quality through the choices we make that are consistent with our values.

◆ VALUE: We're looking at how much value the things we buy actually provide us. When we do this, we also tap into our belief systems and our emotional vitality. The value we get from something is driven by what makes us feel good. We must be aware of our values.

◆ CHOICE: Having money gives us the power to choose from among the things money will buy. We often have more credibility when we have more money. That's how money gives us choices. What we choose to purchase is directed by our personal values, beliefs and points of view.

Why Money Doesn't Equal Happiness

Money doesn't make us happy; it's what we do with our lives that fulfills us or not. Money allows us to manage the quality, value and choices that come into our lives. When we do that successfully, we are financially vital. We have to define what quality and choices we want in order to know how much financial fitness we want to have.

When we think about the things that help manage quality, value and choice what we're really doing is managing our vital signs - just like with Physical Vitality.

The Vital IGN of Money

Some vital signs for Financial Viability are:

◆ Tax Liability   ◆ Cash Flow   ◆ Professional Credibility/Integrity
◆ Gross Income   ◆ Savings   ◆ Length of Time Working
◆ Net Income   ◆ Debt   ◆ Long Term Savings
◆ Credit Profile   ◆ Net Worth ◆ Monthly Sufficiency Factors
◆ Investment Income ◆ Insurance   ◆ Working Years Until
                              Risk   Retirement Age

These indicate our vitality in the financial domain. In Physical Vitality, it is up to us to take responsibility for our body's health and longevity. In Financial Vitality, it is expected that we take care of our money's ability to keep up with our life. If we are Financially Vital, in a sense it doesn't matter how much money we make. These vital signs really represent how much life we live with the money that comes into our life. How much do we enjoy our lives?

A Life Worth Living Is What Gives Value To Money

If a woman has Family as a high value in life and is a millionaire, but never spends time with her family, then having more money didn't give her more value. She is not Financially Vital. If a man is poor and cannot pay his bills - but he has plenty of time for family - then he, too, is not Financially Vital. In many ways it's a balancing act.

What really matters is how and why we live in the presence of money. How much value are we able to appreciate with the money in our lives? Our lives have to be worth living. That is what gives value to having money.

If the most important thing to us is spending time with our family, then we want to make sure we have the kind of money in our lives that will help us do that - at least at an acceptable level.

Money Is Energy

Money is not just something we earn and spend on things. It's a kind of energy in our lives. Using it negatively will produce those effects in our financial life. The same happens if we use it irresponsibly - we produce more of that same irresponsible energy and so on. For example, you can create a lot of stress (not to mention bad credit) by racking up credit card debt when you don't have the cash to pay for what you bought. The problem is that most of us live miles away from the city of Financial Vitality. We don't have a clue about money as a form of energy.

For so long, we have let financial institutions such as insurance companies and credit card companies run our financial lives. We've trusted them with our money - our energy - and we're drained because we don't know what we're doing with our own money/energy. We have the idea that someone else will take care of our energy. They'll help us when we're short of it, cover us when we're in a medical emergency and assist us when we retire.

Who's In Charge Of Your Energy?

Think again. No one else can always have our best financial interests in mind. Who should? That's right, OURSELVES. Once again, the responsibility is ours. It's ours, not just because it's our money, but because the flow of energy in our lives will work better for us if we learn to manage and master money.

Yes, by all means, engage the services of accountants, enrolled agents, bankers, and certified financial planners. However, *we* must take full responsibility for the role money plays in our lives. If we don't know how to manage the vital signs of our financial life, we can turn to those financial professionals who will teach us. It's OK to use the services of the money wizards as long as we delegate effectively and manage the authority we delegate.

Financial Training

Take one vital sign at a time and focus primarily on it. Work with people who have mastery in that specific area. In Physical Vitality, we might hire a fitness trainer to help us get in shape. In Financial Vitality, we might go to a financial planner who helps us structure our earnings, investments and our savings. Ultimately, we can structure our life so that the money we have in our lives gives us the most value, choices and quality.

The Mirror Of Money

We must live our lives in a way that has meaning for us, then go on and create the money that will support what we love doing. Through our living, we can tell how much life we produce with our money. Money is a feedback system of reading how effective our contribution is to the life energy of the planet. The more we contribute in a healthy way, the more money we will make to support our lives.

Making More

Now that we know the meaning of money in our life, the next obvious question is, "How can we make more money?" There are millions of ways people can do that within the context of their life-work. It's up to the creativity of each person. (See chapter on Professional Vitality). We might also want to ask ourselves, "If we could have all the money we needed, what would we do with our lives? What would be important to us if money wasn't an issue? What would make life worth living?"

The answers to these questions will help us see what has value to us personally. Then we can look at what degree our current financial resources allow us to experience that value - and for how long. From there, we can develop a plan or goal and act responsibly according to our values.

One of the best financial books I have ever read is Suze Orman's *The 9 Steps to Financial Freedom*, ISBN 0-517-70791-8.

PART THREE

Being There, Getting On With Life

13

MASTERY AND COMPLETE VITALITY

Now we know about life in the seven cities of vitality. In this chapter we'll learn the five levels of mastery and how to identify our level of mastery in each area. We'll also discover what to do in the areas where we might need improvement.

Let's say, for example, we are frustrated with the sport of tennis. What are our reasons? Most likely it's because we're not very good players or we don't know all the rules of tennis. The more we practice and understand the rules, the better our game gets and the more we enjoy playing.

The Game Of Life

The same idea applies to the sport of life. If we don't know how to eat nutritiously, exercise properly, learn continuously, or behave responsibly and consciously, then we won't know how to live with complete vitality.

If we don't know how to live with complete vitality, then we are probably not enjoying life to its fullest possibility. The more we practice and learn the rules for living vitally, the better we'll get at this life long game.

Becoming a Champion In Complete Vitality

Our goal is to cultivate ourselves until we're winners. Once we're consistent winners, we continue to improve in every area of the sport until we're champions. After the season championship, we continue to practice and refine our skills until the next season and the process of life goes on and on.

Being champions in Complete Vitality means that we have gotten so competent in each of the seven aspects of Vitality, we can wear the title of master. We have earned our black belts in our area of expertise. We know much of what there is to know about our "sport" and we practice and teach what we know.

Some people are born to become champions in some areas even if they lose a few games. Some of us have to work hard for a single win. Sometimes, if we don't win a game after having worked so hard, we might make the mistake of believing we are no good. When we make that mistake, we may lose our self-esteem. We may even buy into the feeling that we are losers in life.

Vitality And Self-Esteem

We sometimes forget to distinguish between who we are and what we are capable of doing. We forget that our values (i.e., being an honest person) and our competence (i.e., being good at tennis) are two separate issues.

Just because we may not be winners in a game does not mean we are bad people. [And] being a good person doesn't automatically make one good at the game of Complete Vitality either. It is important to understand our own level of competence in each area of Complete Vitality. Then we can decide what we might want to work on without getting stuck in a rut while on the quest for Complete Vitality.

Getting More Out Of Life

If it is important for our happiness in life to play tennis well, then we'll need to do what it takes to make that happen. The same goes for living with vitality. To achieve complete vitality, we need to give ourselves permission to live, learn and grow into fully empowered beings with mastery in any and every area of life.

It is crucial that we get rid of our emotional baggage of anger, anxiety, fear and frustration. Then we can begin the process of becoming masters of the vitality of our physical, psychological, emotional, spiritual, intellectual, professional and financial lives.

Mastery and Complete Vitality

But how do we become masters of complete vitality? It's quite clear what a tennis player might do. He would probably get with a coach, learn the techniques of playing great tennis and practice several hours a day, season after season.

In life, a first step toward mastery is to understand our level of competence in the seven different areas. If we haven't achieved mastery in complete vitality, then where are we, and how do we achieve mastery in each area?

The following are the five levels of mastery. Perhaps you'll discover that you are a master in professional vitality, but not even close in spiritual vitality. For each area of your life, look to identify which level most applies to you.

It is crucial to remember that to master anything, we must start at the first level and work through all the steps. People who try to take shortcuts are setting themselves up for failure, every time.

Level 1 . . . The Novice

We are novices if we are acknowledged new students of any discipline. In the particular subject at hand, we are unconsciously, incompetent because we don't know what we don't know. We don't even know the questions to ask about the things we don't know. No one expects us to know very much because we have said, "I am a novice at this activity."

As a novice tennis player, we might not have a clue about how to hold a racquet. As a novice in spiritual vitality, we may not realize our connectedness or disconnectedness with the universe.

Eighty percent of our job as a novice is to make sure we accumulate information about our topic of interest. We must begin to understand the rules and relationships of the area in which we are seeking competence.

Level 2 . . . The Amateur

Once we have reached the point where information gathering is no longer crucial to participation, we have become amateurs. Now we are consciously incompetent, because we can at least acknowledge what we don't know. We are expected to have some ability in the subject, even if we are not very good at it. We have a fairly good idea about things though, because we have seen, experimented with, or heard of most things to do with it.

As an amateur guitar player we might go to an "open-mike-night" at a bar or volunteer to play for the girl scout's campfire. As an amateur in physical vitality we have a sense of how to eat right and exercise regularly.

The most important thing for us as amateurs, is to spend 80% of our time and energy practicing and getting coaching (see Coaching in Resources Chapter) to help us refine our practice sessions. We want to internalize, memorize and understand the big picture of what we are trying to accomplish.

Level 3 . . . The Rookie

When we have the big picture and we have decided to commit to learning and developing a high level of competence in our area, we have become a rookie. We have conscious competence, because we have a larger awareness about the thing in which we are skilled. We think about the decisions we make as we take action to create a big picture.

As rookie baseball players, we know how to play the game about as well as a pro. We just haven't had the experience of doing it in front of thousands of fans. As a rookie in financial vitality, we might get experience by doing the accounting for the family business.

Our job as rookies is to spend 80% of our time connecting each facet of our skill to our big picture and creating a larger vision for ourselves. Continue to be coached. It is essential for rookies to have more than one coach so they can experience several different points of view and areas of expertise.

Level 4 . . . The Pro

As a pro, we have almost reached mastery, except that our knowledge is still internalized. We make sure our responses and behavior abide by the rules and regulations of the particular activity. At this point, we are somewhere between the conscious competent and the unconscious competent. The choices we make and the actions we take are almost automatic.

Our job as pro, is to spend eighty percent of our time developing connection and language communication between us and people who have different areas of expertise than our own. They have important knowledge to add to the accomplishment of our goal and vice versa.

For example, as technicians with a product to sell, we need to bring in people who are experts in sales. That way we can bridge the gap between what we create and how we get paid for it. We also might need accountants, attorneys, financial planners, managers, etc., if we are not competent in these areas.

In evolving toward mastery, we discover how to externalize our knowledge. As a pro in intellectual vitality, for example, we would teach what we know to a wider and more diverse audience.

Hence the word, professor. We know our art at every level of our fiber and being. We are developing the language required to teach our skill to the next generation of novices who are now looking for enlightenment through mastery in our field.

Level 5 . . . The Master

As a pro, we may have taught our knowledge in some straightforward manner. The difference with mastery is now we can convey the life lessons we have acquired to the next generation as coach, consultant, teacher, enlightened one. Who we have become is because of the mastery we have achieved through our art or skill.

For example, as a master of a Martial Art, we have achieved more than an ability to defend ourselves. What is more important is that we have attained a level of awareness about life, a knowledge of our inner selves, a recognition of our purpose on the planet and an acceptance of our responsibility as a human being.

With mastery in Professional Vitality, we are the heads of departments, businesses and industries. We have a knack for intuitively knowing the outcome of a project or challenge, just by looking at some small element of the beginning.

There is no hard and fast way to achieve mastery. Mastery assumes a level of maturity, competence, awareness and communication. Mastery carries a special wisdom that our society has difficulty recognizing. Conventional psychology leaves off at recognizing the level of unconscious competent or pro. Mastery takes us far beyond this understanding to an awareness with which we are vaguely familiar. Perhaps this is why it is such a challenge for us to understand the process of mastering vitality.

An Evolving Process

Imagine a world full of people who have reached mastery in the complete vitality process. As life is forever ongoing, we must remember that the mastery of complete vitality is not a destination, plateau or end. It is a state of being that we achieve and then maintain while on our life's journeys. It is an evolving process.

In our quest for complete vitality we must peel off the layers of limitations that we have put on ourselves, our abilities, our ideas of who we are and our perceptions of the quality of life that is available to us.

As you can very well imagine, everyone's path to mastering vitality is going to be as different as the individual. In the next chapter, I share with you some ideas that I always keep in mind and that I never forget in my own quest for complete vitality.

14

LIMITLESS
BOUNDARIES

Completely vital people have a set of personal rules to live by. No two people are the same, so their personal parameters will differ widely. When you come across people who you think are completely vital, ask them about the three or four things they always do and several key things they never do. Here is my own success system for living with complete vitality.

My "Always" List

1. Evolve

Always plan to evolve. There is no one event that will occur someday to make everything you want magically happen. Whatever is going on with you right now is preparing and empowering you for what will be going on tomorrow, next month, next year. Do not resist change — Grow with it and live through it. Capitalize on the lessons you are learning. Make your life better because of change. Count on change.

2. Trends

Keep your eyes and ears open to new ideas and trends. Find out what people need and are looking for. As a business, you can restructure and repackage your product and service to respond to the current needs of your clients and customers. Keep learning new languages, new ways of doing things and new systems of thought. If you do, you will never be caught unconscious or unaware of upcoming changes and the challenges inherent within them. By staying in tune with the times, you will always have a job, somewhere with someone.

3. Moderate

Keep things in perspective. The fate of the whole world is not wrapped around the outcome of any one thing, any one person, or any one event. Maintain high moral principles and live by them. Do not be a martyr to only one way of achieving your dream. Be open to course corrections and to counsel from those you admire and respect. Take care of your body, so that you can be present to enjoy the process of life and the fruit of your dedication and hard work. Be willing to take your own advice before you give it. Ask permission to speak candidly before you tell the truth directly. Be diplomatic and compassionate. For everything there is a "right time" to act.

4. Respect

Empower the people around you, but do not be dysfunctional. Acknowledge something unique and special about the people you meet.

When it is time to complete with people, be complete mutually and without remorse. Wish them well, even if you disagree on major issues. Respect others even if you don't like them or what they do.

My "Never" List

1. Dependent

Never pack more than you can carry and run with. Be self-reliant. Do not make others responsible for your choices in life. Always be willing to take full responsibility for what is important to you. Unload excess baggage and emotional garbage.

2. Ungrateful

Never make the mistake of diminishing the value of the contribution that other people are able to make to your life. Your job is just as important as the job of the people you work for and who work for you. You need their commitment and competence and they need your excellence and vision. As people, we exist in an interdependent social eco-system. Everyone is significant. Do not discount anyone.

3. Money-Hungry

Never make money more important than anything else. Money is a by-product of contribution to the planet through service. The greater and more efficient the contribution, the greater the reward. Reward and financial security is nice, but you must have health and family in order to appreciate quality. Do not be rich and lonely, without the love of friends and family — that is no life at all.

4. Give Up

Never give up on yourself. You have to come through for you no matter what. Above all, love yourself enough to believe in you. The reason you have a dream is to keep yourself focused on what you are capable of.

An "Always" and "Never" list is all about limitless boundaries. It's the success system you have for life. Make a list for yourself. Look for the things you love and hate. Constructively write down rules to create the things you love and avoid the things that don't work for you. It becomes your own personal ten commandments.

15

CHOOSING COMPLETE VITALITY

A Version Of The Elephant Story

There were once five blind sons. Each was assigned to take care of a particular part of the family elephant. One evening at dinner, they were all arguing about what an elephant was really like. Son #1 cared for the trunk of the elephant and insisted an elephant was like a big pipe which made a trumpeting noise. Son #2 cared for the ears and knew for sure that an elephant was like two leather flags blowing in the breeze. Son #3 cared for the legs and argued that the animal was like four great, moving tree trunks. Son #4 cared for the belly and said that it was obviously like a giant melon floating just above the ground. Son #5 cared for the tail and said an elephant is like a rope swishing flies.

The verbal conflagration went on. Each insisted that they were absolutely correct and that the others were out of their minds. Finally, the wise father who could SEE the big picture very well said, "My sons, you are all right and you are all wrong. Each of you is only aware of the part of the elephant you attend. If each of you were to change places with the others, you would know, without a doubt, that the others were correct — and that your views, indeed, have a basis in fact."

Just because their account is different than yours, does not make one version correct and another incorrect or baseless. Before you refute or discount the truth from anyone else's point of view, be sure to spend a year or two learning what they know and seeing what they see. Then you will know the truth for yourself."

Tunnel Vision Syndrome

The "absolutely right and absolutely wrong brothers" are our conventional medical and allied health professionals with all their specialties. This story reflects those health professionals who think their way is the only way to be healthy and whole.

They have all chosen to excel in only one vital aspect of the mastery required to achieve and maintain quality of life and peace of mind, body, and spirit.

Many of those professionals and practitioners, like the blind brothers, reached the level of competence of "PRO." Then some of their inflated egos got in the way and they stopped asking questions; they stopped learning from their masters; they stopped considering the possibility that there was another correct point of view that could broaden their own. They stopped respecting each other's rights and privileges; they even tried to ridicule and exterminate each other several times. They are all right AND they are often wrong.

The Right To Choose

Some of our health professionals tried to monopolize our attention and confuse us with inaccuracies and partial truths. Some of them tried to take away our right to choose. Some of our well-meaning experts tried to make us feel that they know what is good for us and they are only trying to do what is in our best interests.

Sorry folks, not even God tries to take away our right to choose. No matter what our experts say, we can choose how we want to live a healthy and vital existence.

Here is another inalienable principle of life:

No institution where there is power or profit involved acts purely in the best interests of its constituents or customers.

This is true in politics, religion, in every business and in education - it is just that way. The only way to ensure the quality of your own life is for you to personally go through the process of ensuring it.

I am suggesting that the only way for you to achieve mastery in complete vitality is to go through each step toward mastery in a deliberate way. Make sure you are the one in charge of your own mission toward vitality. The choices are for you to make.

We must make sure however, that the possibilities for our choices are available to make. Already, many of the holistic methods toward complete vitality are extinct or on the endangered species list. That may mean more effort and attention on our part. No matter what, we have to let our providers, elected officials and product developers know what we want made available to us. We must protect our privileges and rights to choose the kind of health care we really want.

Choosing to be completely vital can be an uphill battle. Let us assume there are no adversaries at this point. There is no health care industry giving you inaccurate information, no commercials giving you poor choices from which to choose, no politicians working for the various interests to pass laws that increase our dependence on the system, no friends telling us we are crazy for considering holistic ways to respond to health challenges.

Now, we are left with hundreds of books, tapes, sciences, gimmicks and experts who are trying to tell us, "My way is the best, right and only way there ever was. [And] you should trust me because I know better than you and I have your best interests in mind."

Don't give in to your confusion and feelings of powerlessness. Now that you have vitality as an ideal, you have a better idea of how to start achieving it. That leads us to: THE ULTIMATE QUESTION:

How Do I Become Completely Vital?

In the case of our elephant story, it would be like asking the elephant for the real answers to our health and lifestyle concerns. [But] in reality there is no elephant to ask, no wise dad to straighten it out for us. We are stuck with the challenge of finding the answers for ourselves. Hence you have this book and the many others that teach us about our wholeness.

The Simple Answer To The Ultimate Question

You cannot know all your answers right now. You figure it out along the way. You have to trust your inner voice to guide you. When you are "there" you know it, because you are healthy, content, stress-neutral, financially comfortable, spiritually grounded, and emotionally balanced with a fulfilling recreational and social life.

The Real Answer -
Seven Steps To Complete Vitality

Using a journal, a piece of paper, or your computer, write down and complete the following thoughts:

STEP ONE: "When I am physically vital, on a physical level the following things will be true about me - (see chapter 6)

A. I will look like.....
B. I will be able to.....

The way I will feel about that is....."

STEP TWO: "When I am emotionally spiritually vital spiritual level.....(see chapter 8, 9)

A. This will look like.....
B. I will be able to....

The way I will feel about that is....."

STEP THREE: "When I am mentally emotional vital (see chapter 7, 10)

A. This will look like....
B. I will be able to....

The way I will feel about that is....."

STEP FOUR: "When I am financially and professionally vital (includes career, your relationship with money, and ???) (see chapter 11, 12)

A. This will look like.....
B. I will be able to.....

The way I will feel about that is....."

Two Secrets About Achieving Complete Vitality

◆ It is only possible to recognize complete vitality after we can articulate it.

◆ We can only articulate complete vitality in terms of what we can or intend to be able to do with it.

When you have your goals and intentions articulated, you can move on to:

STEP FIVE: Choose the first area on which you want to focus your intentions.

STEP SIX: Look for people who are already at the PRO or MASTERY (see chapter 13) level in that area. Perhaps they may be in the business of teaching and coaching individuals in that area already.

They may even be your current friends or people you can add to your circle of friends.

STEP SEVEN: Practice, ask for guidance, practice again. Keep a written journal of what you discover, learn and feel. Practice until you feel you have it right enough for you.

Pretend that you are a novice at this point, collecting information from anybody and everybody who has an answer and a point of view. Their ideas will give you insight into your own sense of what is right for you. Only you can know in the end that you chose the right thing, because your life will work for you and you will be at peace with the result.

Identifying Your Truth in Complete Vitality

How your truth represents itself in your life may turn out to be a hybrid of everyone else's truth you have heard. That is okay, because now it is your truth and yours is different from everyone else's.

A person's answers are only one set of answers from one point of view. They are still right (from their end of the elephant). What they say or recommend is only right if you try it and it works for you.

While on your quest, what works for you may not work for the next person and vice versa. Always gauge their results with your own goals and take their suggestions in light of your personal experience. Remember, you must choose for yourself what works.

Do not pass judgment on other people [personally] or hold them hostage [morally] to their level of mastery [professionally]. As for our ailing medical industrial complex, bear in mind that there are mostly good, caring, compassionate professionals working within a system that needs to change.

Malpractice lawsuits won't change a bad system. Neither will defensive medicine. Health care coverage is not the solution either. Having more of it merely puts gasoline on a fire that will kill us all or bankrupt us (or both!). Managed care may get worse before it gets better.

Being Part of the Solution

With all your professionals in every field of expertise, pay gratefully in cash for empowerment. With placating, uninformative or condescending professionals, don't return or make it crystal clear - in advance - that you are paying for the empowering answers to some questions you have. You expect courtesy and direct answers in plain, understandable language. Get their agreement with those terms or try the caring, compassionate, informative professional down the street.

For the record, I am not a medical professional or any type of primary care provider in the system. I am only one person working on the elephant. I am making a recommendation about how I would and do handle my health care and lifestyle improvement professionals. I am not - and never have been - in the diagnosis business. You should see the people who are trained to make diagnoses, when it is appropriate.

You have the right to choose what you want. You have the responsibility to uphold your right to dictate the quality of vitality you want to enjoy. You can - and should - go to everybody and anybody who might have an answer to your questions or a solution to your problems.

You are the one who decides what level of vitality is right for you.

I recommend, however, that since you have to work hard anyway; choose to work diligently toward creating a life of vitality, longevity and self-reliance. That way, you'll be able to enjoy doing whatever else it is that you want to accomplish in life.

16

THE FUTURE OF LONGEVITY

For as long as we can imagine, people have been searching for a way to prolong life and youthfulness. Vitality, by definition, is the ability to create life from energy. Living with complete vitality is the secret to longevity and quality of life.

However, we've got to consider the effects vitality will have on our future. Think about this: a life with vitality means no disease. There's nothing to "naturally" die from. The only causes of death are accidents, homicide, suicide, unwitting exposure to lethal toxins and acts of war or terrorism.

Sounds great, but longevity has its price. For a lot of us the price isn't even something we can imagine right now. Did you know that the body is capable of living 120-140 years and perhaps more?

Looking At A Longer Life

If we start living that long with excellent health and quality of life, just think how differently our society will have to function. For example:

1. How do we plan financially for an extra 80 years of longevity?

2. What will the average retirement age become? Instead of 65, maybe it's 100.

3. How do we plan our careers?

4. How do we plan for family life?

5. What would replace our current systems of health care, insurance, social security... if we are so vital we don't need them anymore?

Planning for the result of complete vitality is like a couple who, upon announcing their engagement, start putting away college money for their first child. People who decide to live vitally need to plan for their longevity.

We have to refigure all the issues surrounding "old age," retirement and maturity. We can start by answering for ourselves these kinds of questions:

1. How long do you think you will live given your current health care maintenance program?

2. If it were possible to live with dignity and quality for an indefinite time, how long would you like to live?

I did a small survey recently in which I asked those questions of 100 of my clients. Of five individuals over 50 who responded to my small study, one could see himself living to age 85. Another could only imagine living to 125-150. The other three said they would like to live forever, if possible. One explained, "I feel like I have finally figured some things out for myself... if I could start here and know that I have at least twice my lifetime ahead of me, then I would really enjoy life. I would have my money, wisdom, time and energy to enjoy new things, new friends, activities, travel, etc.

How Old Is Old?

Not long ago, the Baby Boom generation thought fifty was old, and seventy was synonymous with decrepit and senile. Now eighty seems old. However, all around us are more examples and role models of wisdom, maturity and fun... at 60, 70, 80 and even 100. Almost nothing will be the same for us at 90 as it is for 90 year-olds today.

Can we imagine what our lives will be like when we are twice or thrice our current age? I am suggesting that we take a serious look at some possibilities. [And] there are three major areas to consider:

1. Defining and ensuring quality of life with longevity.

2. Affordability and variety of health care and body maintenance.

3. Retirement planning for an extra eighty years.

We must think about preparing for this future now. We don't want to end up having to choose the quality of our future by default. I am not suggesting we need to come up with the "right" answers at this time. I am implying that we will be better off if we start expanding our minds to include new possibilities beyond imagination.

Vitality Has No Age

We may need to update our vision about what life will be like when we are vital and mature. We live in a country that disrespects and disregards the value of maturity and wisdom. Age is not a measure of vitality. Complete vitality is a measure of the life force that is able to manifest in our mind, body and spirit.

Longevity can be miserable without vitality and quality of life. We must make sure we take care of our bodies as though we intend to have them for at least another 100 years.

The Conflict With Our Bodies

In this new age, ever more of us find that our spirits and minds are geared for immortality. [But] after years of abuse, our bodies are programmed for breakdown and illness at an early age.

We have a conflict of directions here. We try to get quality of life through money, material things and the different groups or activities in which we participate. [But] we become unable to enjoy these things with longevity because of the poor choices and habits we have about health, well-being and personal fulfillment. If there is no vitality in our physical bodies, vitality in any other area is impossible.

We must stop neglecting our bodies and tune in to its real needs for vitality.

The Future For The 'Me' Generation

Baby Boomers are now discovering that life is not over at fifty or sixty—[But] just a new beginning. It is almost like being reborn. In our futures, retirement is likely to be cyclical. We retire from a profession or livelihood only to take time to educate ourselves for yet another profession and so on. Our lives are likely to include a nice balance of education, profession and enjoyment throughout the years. (For more on this see: www.agewave.com).

Why Should We Live Longer?

Perhaps no one knows exactly how to live forever with quality in every situation. Many of us know no one who has lived long enough to be an example of a future of longevity we would want for ourselves.

Why do we like the idea of longer lives? When we have quality, dignity and energy, we want longevity. Then we can enjoy more life. We think there will be more possibilities for us as time goes by. We want more time to learn from the mistakes of our youth. We want to live with the same kind of energy, but with the wisdom and maturity of years of experience.

We want more time and ability to make our contribution to the planet. Without our physical health, none of this is possible.

Choose to live with complete vitality if you have plans for yourself and the world. Choose to live vitally if you want to continue evolving and mastering life's lessons. Choose to live with vitality if you want to improve the quality of life for your great, great, great grandchildren. Choose to live vitally if you have a way to restore health to our ecology, economy, families or social systems. The planet and its people need you to succeed with your plans and dreams for the future.

17

INTEGRATIVE MEDICINE - A COMPETITIVE EDGE

Many holistic healers have had a hard time being taken seriously in their professions. For generations, the conventional medical industry has used its powerful associations to undermine the contributions of holistic healers. The industry has done a good job turning average, otherwise open-minded people into skeptics about holistic healing.

Using The Media

One of the medical industry's best aggressive tactics is through the media. While the media thinks it's posing as a watchdog for the people, often it ends up acting as a henchman for conventional medicine. Over the years I've watched as journalists have ruthlessly interrogated, then professionally crucified holistic practitioners.

The media cleverly sets up the 10-minute story as an inquisition of holistic practitioners. Using bad lighting in a hurried atmosphere, they interrogate a practitioner like this: "Isn't it true that you...(insert accusation)...? Why should we believe your claims that your stuff can produce these results, which experts say are impossible? Where are your scientific studies?" It goes on until the unprepared healer says something incriminating, then it's over with.

Then they counter that in an interview with an "expert." In a nice close-up shot, they ask, "Dr. Expert, how can so-and-so get away with this? How can we guard against being taken advantage of by jerks like this?"

These days, a growing forty-three percent of people seeking medical help also consider holistic solutions. People, discouraged by conventional medical advice and practices, sometimes fall prey to unscrupulous phonies who talk a good story and do a good dance, but don't know what they're doing professionally. This does a great disservice to practitioners who DO practice legitimately. It also does a disservice to potential clients and patients who may never get to benefit from the art and service of a true holistic practitioner.

Uncovering Quacks

It is good when journalists expose the impostors - and they should be commended when they do. However, discrediting an entire holistic profession is hardly accurate or responsible journalism.

Journalists often focus 90% of our attention on the three percent at the bottom of the holistic practitioner's success curve. They leave us to assume that all holistic practices and claims are bogus.

Uncovering Journalists

As we look at news segments like these, it is wise to ponder the following questions:

1. Why is this story really being done?
2. In whose best interest is the angle of the story reported?
3. Who is the "good guy" and "bad guy" here?
4. If this were an advertisement, what is being sold?

Often a news piece is no different from an infomercial. This would explain many biases. It is important to qualify the nature of the health, medical or news programs - even commercials. Don't let yourself be swayed by incomplete, biased news programming. Notice how much time is put into offering a fair representation of the practitioner, the science he or she applies and the percentage success rate he and his colleagues have with their clients.

Following The Witch Hunters

The enormous power of the conventional medical industrial complex can crush all challengers to its professional and financial interests. [But] only if we blindly believe they're acting in our best interests and let them go unchecked.

We are trained to see only what "they" want us to see. If we find a conventional medical person doing questionable practices we think, "This one doctor is bad and should be put out of business."

When a holistic practitioner becomes the subject of scrutiny or scandal, we tend to think, "All healers of this discipline are unscientific crooks practicing 'quack' medicine. They should be burned at the stake!" Which is exactly what happened in the old days - they literally killed off holistic healers by naming them witches and scaring the public. These days, the hunters prefer the more civil approach of condemnation through litigation, the media, and public brainwashing.

The Art Of Science

The reputation of holistic healing would gain more widespread acceptance if its practitioners would defend themselves more scientifically and comprehensively. In this regard, holistic healers have much to learn from the power brokers and orchestrators of our medical industrial complex.

Instead of presenting their science like an art, holistic healers need to present their art like a science. They need to look and speak like the most eloquent physicists who ever lived, so there can be no doubt about the rightness of what they do.

As it is, healers are often the worst at explaining what they do in a way that can be clearly understood. Here are my recommendations to practitioners and healers who wish to position themselves as leaders and competent authorities in the various fields of holistic health.

Do The Scientific Homework

Get every piece of data from every related study that has ever been done anywhere in the world. Collect articles. Check facts. Don't assume you are so unique in your practice, that you are the first person who ever thought of such a great idea. Look for other people who are doing similar work in your town or somewhere else.

If you cannot find scientific studies in your field, bring in some knowledgeable scientists and do one yourself. Have your scientific records on hand. Be prepared to go public with your findings. Use scientific methods, speak authoritatively and use plain English. Create two versions of your science - one for the scientific community and one for the lay person.

Perfect Your Presentation

Hire speech coaches. Use video feedback so that you are absolutely confident about how and what you say to represent yourself and your healing art. Hire image and wardrobe consultants to ensure that your visual image is impeccable.

You want to look and sound so exquisite that clients and patients want to be healed by you. You want to be so successful and politically correct that other professionals accept and want to be like you. You want them to admire your contribution and aspire to your success.

Hire Good Marketing And Public Relations People

If pet rocks, sushi and TV-evangelism can make zillionaires in this country, you can sell your services and live reasonably well in your town. Your goal must be to position your profession and your art as an ethical, effective and irreproachable system of healing and health achievement.

Make it easy for marketing and public relations people to understand who needs the services you offer. The top three pressing health problems are: affordability, availability and effectiveness. Even if you cannot afford a good marketing consultant, at least expect to become consciously competent at representing and marketing your service through your clients.

Network, Network, Network

Network With Professional Allies

NETWORK #1: Network and ally yourself with others in your profession. Holistic healers tend not to communicate with each other or share tips and ideas about what works for them in their practices. In a sense, we are all trying to be the greatest healer of them all. Bear this in mind - the world is so ill and astray from complete vitality, that there is more than enough work for all healers for several generations.

Create alliances. Join or create associations within your profession. Refer your client's friends in other towns to professionals you know and respect.

Companion Business

NETWORK #2: Network among people who are in companion businesses (which means they offer their services to your same target market). Word-of-mouth networking will build your business and reputation better and faster than the slickest, most expensive advertising. By marketing through people in companion businesses, you will find a set of people who are willing to use your name and refer people to you. If you are not in competition with them and are good at what you do, then it makes them look good in what they do.

Business owners who work in your same market are more likely to hear about the problems of their customers that you could address. For example, I am a massage therapist. My clients are typically people who have high stress jobs or do heavy work, in which they could be injured. The people who are in companion businesses to mine are chiropractic doctors, acupuncturists, colon hygienists, hair stylists and manicurists.

Professional Rivals

NETWORK #3: Network with professionals who might see you as a threat to their business. Most of their viewpoints are based on a lack of information fed to them over the years by people who are unreliable or ill-informed about your science or art. You have the opportunity to update their information and create a professional friend to whom you can refer some of your clients. Learn from them about their profession and art.

In networking, you must become a master at saying what you do, in thirty seconds or less. Use simple sentences or phrases and give three immediate, tangible benefits to your prospects or clients. Any more information is not likely to get transferred. Any more time spent explaining your message is not likely to be regarded at all.

Keep Accurate Client Notes And Records Of Small And Large Breakthroughs

Take photos and/or x-rays to show measurable, visible proof of your work. Get testimonials at the completion of your course of treatments or services to your clients. Keep records in a way that is replicable and simple for laymen to understand. This will be essential for you if you ever find it necessary to substantiate the claims of your service. A good marketing tool is before and after photographs and testimonial letters that show the benefits available through your service.

Keep Accurate Financial Records

Pay your taxes and fees completely, honestly and on time. Have a good enrolled agent, accountant or bookkeeper to make sure your reports, payments and papers are in order and up to date.

Keep A Good Relationship

With The Toughest Lawyer In Your Town

Ask him or her, questions about the reproachability of your statements, claims and methods. Follow your attorney's advice about how to do what you want to do. Learn how to present what you do in a way that will cause you the least amount of anxiety and problems. This is in case you ever have to defend yourself and your profession to the media or a court of law.

Be A Watchdog And Spokesperson For Your Profession

Support legislation that is in your best interest. Write and call your elected officials. Encourage your clients to do the same. Diligently guard your rights to practice your art. No one else will do this for you. Even if you are above reproach, it is the media's perception that can make or break you. Keep your eyes open and keep everyone on their toes.

Always Do Business With The Highest Integrity

Charge fair rates that are competitive with market forces. Make every client a satisfied client or give a fair or full refund. Work as though you expect to have more than 100% success rate with your clients. You cannot afford even one mildly dissatisfied customer. Make it easy to do business with you. Have a simple rate structure that the customer can control to fit their time and financial budget. Become a master at excellent customer service.

Be In The Education And Empowerment Business

Tell your story about how you were led to practice your art. People are inspired by personal testimony. Teach your clients and patients what you know and how you came to those conclusions. Let them know - in simple, repeatable language - why your science works the way it does. Tell them what to teach their friends, family and children. Your strength, credibility and longevity in your profession are what your clients know and can pass on by word of mouth.

People in the holistic health fields have a tough row to hoe - and the industry is making sure we've got an uphill battle. [But] the growing numbers of clients and customers of holistic practitioners are testimony to the fact that we are a needed and important industry. [And] we are making a difference.

18

RESOURCES for Complete Vitality

Complete vitality, as we have discussed in this book, is not the focus of conventional, western medicine. So where do you go for this kind of natural healing and holistic maintenance? Complete vitality services are not something you can go just anywhere to find. What do you do if you have an idea of what you want, but you're not sure where to go, who to call or how to get there? Here is an incomplete list of some healing practices you can turn to as natural alternatives.

Yoo-Hoo- Where Are You?

At first, they may be difficult to find in your community. This loose constellation of talented and often extraordinary practitioners has yet to organize themselves into any strong cohesive force. [But] usually if you find one, they can direct you to practitioners of other forms of complementary holistic healing.

Holistic practitioners may not recognize themselves as part of any new world order of complete vitality. You'll know who they are though, if their professional goal is your empowerment and self-reliance.

Acupuncture/Acupressure

Oriental Medicine umbrellas this form of healing. Using an understanding of the five elements (wind, water, fire, air and earth), acupuncturists and acupressurists can figure out where the body is malfunctioning. Doctors of Oriental Medicine (O.M.D.) Have at least as many hours of practice and study as a graduating medical student.

A series of fourteen nerve pathways, called meridians, link communication between the extremities and the organs of the body. So, various points on the body, ears, hands or feet stimulate certain organs. There are some 3,000 points on the body that work like buttons. The practitioners essentially activate some buttons on the meridians to help the body achieve normalcy and maintain vital energy flow or "chi."

After centuries of research, Oriental Medicine has tremendous value and is extremely effective in many cases. This form of healing is effective for just about anything. Taking into consideration that your mind, body, spirit and environment are interactive forces affecting the Chi energy, practitioners ask questions to begin their diagnosis. What do you eat? How much sleep do you get? How are your bowel movements? What kinds of foods do you crave? They look at your vital signs, tongue, eyes, etc. They often prescribe herbs for normalizing various conditions.

An acupressurist or shiatsu practitioner uses finger pressure on certain meridians and points. An acupuncturist uses needles. The needles feel a bit like flossing your teeth - they don't hurt if you don't move. The thin needles and skilled practitioner, rarely make you bleed. People go to acupuncturists or acupressurists, for anything from cancer to PMS to quitting smoking.

The important thing to remember in any form of healing, is that the person being healed needs to have the will to be healed. In Western medicine, we've been conditioned to believe that taking a pill will cure everything for us. In Chinese medicine, if the person's own will is not present, their healing may not be as effective.

Reviewed by the office of Dr. Sue Y. Lin, O.M.D., ACM Health Center, San Mateo, CA, (650) 579-5792

Applied Kinesiology

This recognized science is an ingenious offspring of a part of Oriental Medicine. It is used as a system of assessment or analysis for practitioners such as chiropractors, sports therapists and body workers.

By pushing or pulling on your arm, leg or fingers a certain way, practitioners test the muscles, not for strength, but for the flow of electro-chemical energy. When all your circuits are working right, the practitioner feels the energy flowing freely. If your body is deficient or something is bad for it, the stimulation to that muscle won't flow and the muscle will test "weak."

Practitioners might put a pill, rock or nutrient (which all vibrate at a certain frequency) in your hand or suggest a certain idea (which is a form of energy) to see if it maintains already open circuits or if it helps make the circuits stronger when muscle-tested. To the uninitiated, it can seem like hocus-pocus. However, this learned skill is a safe, quick and easy method of testing for anything that might be wrong in the body.

Ayurveda

Oriental Medicine is to the Chinese what Ayurveda is to the Indians of the Far East. It's a science, based on sound experiments, that goes back many thousands of years. It too, acknowledges the synchrony of the mind, body, spirit and emotions.

The system uses, among other things, certain exercises like Yoga postures and breathing techniques. You don't just use Ayurveda to heal a sickness, it is a way of life for people who want to maintain vitality. This is true in many well thought-out systems of healing.

In Oriental Medicine, they focus on balancing and maintaining "Chi" energy into the body. In Ayurveda, the goal is to promote the free-flow of energy called "Prana". We have been taught to fix something only when it is broken. Ayurveda is about how to make your body and life whole at all times.

Bodywork Therapy, Somatic Therapy

This way of enhancing the body's ability to achieve wholeness, manipulates the soft tissues. It is different from Chiropractic, Orthopedic or Osteopathic medicine, which manipulate the body's bones and joints.

One distinctive concept in soft tissue manipulation, or deep tissue bodywork, is that just as the brain stores and retrieves data, the body stores and retrieves emotional energy, thoughts, memories and more. Throughout our lives negative emotional energy may get "locked" in our bodies, presenting itself as many physical problems, like poor posture, headaches, chronic pain, poor circulation . . . That negative energy can build on itself like plaque on your teeth. For vitality, receiving bodywork is as important as flossing and brushing your teeth.

There is a national movement to call bodywork, Somatic Therapy. Somo-, meaning body. For the past 25 years, it seems like a new form of Somatic Therapy gets invented every day. More somatic professionals graduate from certification programs every day.

The system of bodywork I've developed is called Reposturing Dynamics. It promotes good posture and flexibility through massage, breathing and a unique series of stretches. A more intensive form of bodywork is Rolfing, which uses pressure and kneading on the muscles and connective tissues.

All forms of bodywork have merit. It just depends on what you want or need at any one time. Different people have different needs at different points in their lives. There's every level of massage from the light, traditional Swedish massage to something deeper like my Reposturing Dynamics, or even Sports Massage.

If your body has never been touched by a professional Somatic practitioner or bodyworker, you might want to start with something easy to receive, like Trager Psychophysical Bodywork or Shiatsu. This can be done through sheets on a fully clothed person. Depending on what you want to achieve, you go to a body worker who does that.

Overall, Somatic Therapies give you a sense of well-being, improved breathing, sleeping, flexibility, energy and a feeling of lightness in your body. This short list could go on and on. Bodywork is that powerful a healing entity.

For a more complete directory of bodywork therapies call Associated Bodywork and Massage Professionals (ABMP) at 1-800-458-2267.

Ask for the Touch Training Directory.

Chiropractic

Your free, uninhibited transmission of energy from the brain to the rest of the body - and vice versa - is maintained by this system of healing. This is done by keeping the specific alignment of the skull and spinal column.

There are some divisions within the profession. While some chiropractic physicians only adjust the spine, others include in their healing: manipulation of soft tissues, the skull and other parts of the body and the spine. It is not a requirement of their practice, but it is within their scope.

Many in the profession are specialists. For example, they may focus on the alignment of the base of the skull and the top two vertebrae. This is based on the idea that if you maintain the alignment of those bones then the rest of the body will align itself. It's worth asking around to see what form of chiropractic might serve you best. By all means, try different types of chiropractic treatment and see for yourself.

In general, Chiropractors are primary care physicians. They treat back problems and more. Even if you have a cold, the thought is that aligning the correct tissues and bones will assist the body's own detoxifying process. One of the concessions made in the truce between the AMA and the Chiropractic profession is the nature of the claims they can make.

Officially they cannot say the many things that happen in the body if you restore and maintain the relationship between the brain and spinal column. However, I can say, as a consumer, I can go to a chiropractor for just about anything, including back problems, headaches or even the flu. They can make medical and holistic referrals when something is out of their professional scope of practice.

Coaching

According to the (now defunct) Professional & Personal Coaching Association (PPCA), coaching is "achieving peak performance without a whistle." It is a professional relationship that enhances a client's ability to effectively focus on learning, making changes, achieving desired goals, and experiencing fulfillment.

Coaches have specialties just like therapists and consultants. Their profession is not designed to heal, as much as it is to enhance and improve. Coaching styles vary depending on the background and training of the coach and needs of the client. Since coaching is a relatively new field, most coaches come from other professions, such as teaching, consulting, and training.

The coach's job is one of skillfully guiding the client toward and along his or her chosen path. By using a coach, clients accelerate and increase positive results in their key result areas: such as business, finance, vitality, personal and professional.

Colon Hygiene

In an ideal and perfect world, our stress-free bodies digest and process only whole, natural, unprocessed, uncooked food that's full of fiber and nutrients. Unfortunately that's not the case. Our digestive system breaks down because we eat foods processed and cooked, with no fiber - not to mention the fact that we don't drink enough water. We also get emotionally affected, locking toxins in our intestines. This may cause unhealthy reactions in our colon.

A professionally done colonic is a safe, hi-tech, clean, odorless way of having an enema. There is a professional called a colon hygienist, who does the colonic irrigations. It's like a roto-rooter for the colon. Nothing goes into the colon except water (although in some circles, coffee or oil enemas are used for specific conditions). A colonic irrigation flushes old stuff out of the colon so it can function normally. Colonics can reawaken stalled peristalsis - the natural rhythm of digestion.

Considering the fact that most of us lead stressful lives and eat processed, cooked food, colonic irrigations are one of the tools for the vital person. Your lifestyle is toxic when you have a lot of stress, eat bad food and drink little water. You should have colonics more often than a person who eats raw, water-rich, fibrous food and is rarely stressed-out. To find a colon hygienist in your area, look in your local yellow pages or the internet under Colon Hygiene. To locate a good one, you may need to ask around.

Environmental Therapies

The way your body heals itself is stimulated through various environmental effects.

Aroma Therapy

We know that certain aromas have different effects on us. The smell of a pizza, flowers, oils, etc., can trigger certain feelings. When working with an aroma therapist, certain smells help promote your healing or maintain your wholeness. More somatic therapists and other healers are adding aromatherapy to their practices every day.

Color Therapy

Certain colors affect the brain. There is a scientific art dedicated to the study of the influence that colors have on us. With the current research, we will see it used ever more. Specific colors will not only influence healing, but also change our moods. It's long been known that pink walls in a prison make inmates less violent. Often women in business wear red to convey more power when they negotiate deals. Products are more appealing to us if they are in certain colors. If you want to enhance a particular aspect of your personality, promote healing or stimulate a business environment, change the colors around you.

Feng Shui

Pronounced "Fung-Shway," it is the art of art of optimizing the life-giving, life-sustaining, energy in a room, a building, or a piece of property. It is different from interior design, or architectural design. Feng Shui experts look for the natural lines in the geometry of the space or land to enhance to enhance the potential for maximum aliveness and essential harmony.

You can use Feng Shui principles almost anywhere. Experts suggest using various accessories and the arrangements of objects to improve the effect of light, heat, sound, traffic flow, and air flow in a living or work space.

Hydro Therapy

Water is known as the ultimate solvent - it can even cut through rocks. Simply using water to wash or soak the body can feel very healing - as in a bath or shower. A Jacuzzi is a water treatment tool, meant for easing tension and relaxing muscles. In ice form, water is used to cool burn victims. It flushes the body's cells of toxins when we drink it. Colonic Irrigation is also a form of Hydro Therapy. Basically, it is using water as a curative.

Probably one of the most enjoyable bodywork sessions I've ever had was in water, using a technique called "watsu". Watsu is a hybrid of shiatsu or accupuncture and gentle stretching while being supported by my Watsu practitioner in a large warm pool. If this appeals to you at all, call the Worldwide Aquatic Bodywork Association at (707) 987-3801 and find a Watsu Practitioner near you.

Light Therapy

Light is a form of energy that measures by frequency, intensity and quantity. It affects the brain. Regular florescent lights are not good for study and work because they flicker at an annoying frequency for the brain. Incandescent lights have a warming affect. Lights of different hues bring out certain moods. The effect of lights on an audience can be dramatically noticed at a music concert. Pay attention to lighting as a major contributor to your wholeness and vitality.

Oxygen Therapy

According to some scientific philosophies, a disease-causing organism cannot exist in an oxygen-rich environment. So if you super-oxygenate the body, these diseases go away. Breathing is one way to do this - the purpose behind Breath Therapy. Drinking oxygenated water helps to neutralize the effects of toxins present in the body. Further, it helps to oxygenate the blood and body tissues.

Sound Therapy

The same idea as color therapy applies here. Music therapists use certain tones to promote healing. Throughout the ages indigenous cultures have used sound in the form of chanting mantras, psalms, and hymns to invoke ones deity and quicken their inner spirit. Healers may use sound in the form of music, or just the tones of different frequencies to enhance therapy or to promote a specific effect.

Graphotherapy

Applied Graphotherapy is a gentle science designed for personal growth. It takes handwriting analysis to the next level and says that, changing your handwriting can change your life.

The handwriting of an individual indicates and reflects who that person is and what their beliefs and attitudes are all about. By intentionally altering specific handwriting components, formations and patterns, different neurological input to the brain occurs. Over a short period of time this stimuli reflects positive changes in the personality, attitudes and belief system of the writer, thus allowing them to pursue their dreams, and achieve their goals.

Graphotherapy is a simple non-threatening tool that puts the capability of change literally into the hands of the individual.

A definitive book on the application of graphotherapy is 'Change Your Handwriting, Change Your Life' by Vimala Rodgers, ISBN #0-89087-693-2. The Spanish Edition is 'Cambia Tu Escritura Para Cambiar Tu Vida', ISBN #84-7953-168-1. This is not a textbook, but a book that can be used by anyone who wants to know who they really are.

Provided by   Dr. Marilyn Carmona
                 San Mateo, CA
                 (650) 342-3452

Herbology

This is the study of how different herbs act biochemically on the system. Many different healing methods use herbs as part of their prescriptions. It is a very ancient science. People have been using herbs as medicines and preparations for thousands of years. In recent history, someone figured out how to synthesize the active ingredient in some medicinal herbs. It's really the root of our modern pharmaceuticals.

A person who is an herbalist knows how herbs affect the body just as a Western medical doctor knows the effects of pharmaceuticals. Unprocessed, unsynthesized herbs often vibrate at a higher frequency, energetically, than pharmaceutical preparations. Your body is more likely to more readily recognize the herbs as something that can be easily processed by the body, so it will use them faster, easier and with fewer side effects, than most laboratory preparations.

Homeopathy

Homeopathy is the use of medicines that come from natural substances such as plants, herbs and minerals to help the body heal itself. These medicines are used instead of conventional drugs. Homeopathy sees the signs of illness in a person as being a result of something in the body not working right. Our bodies have the ability to respond to this and heal themselves. For example, a fever helps the body kill bacteria which may cause illness. Therefore, rather than being something that is caused by a person being sick, a fever is really helping the person get well.

Homeopathic medicines are used to speed up this process, and to work in connection with the body's natural responses to help the person get well. By using homeopathic medicines instead of conventional drugs, the person's overall health and general well-being are improved. Homeopathic therapies have been used with good results for over 200 years. Professionals who are Certified Homeopaths have studied a rigorous program of disease and proper treatment with natural substances.

Provided by   Dr. Nicole Cherok
San Mateo, CA
(650) 348-4262

Hypnotherapy

In Hypnotherapy, a deep state of relaxation is achieved through focused attention. While in this trance-like state, the unconscious mind is highly receptive to new perspectives and ideas. The use of imagery and positive suggestions at this time can help a client imagine and actually experience herself in the future, as she desires to be. This makes the changes she wants in her life happen much faster and with less resistance, as a result of the hypnosis experience.

www.eastendhealth.com/glossary.asp

In the clinical use of hypnosis,the subject's powers of consciousness are mobilized and subconscious memories and perceptions are brought into consciousness. Heightened responsiveness to suggestions and commands, suspension of disbelief with lowering of critical judgements, the potential of alteration in perceptions, motor control,or memory in response to suggestions and the subjective exierence of responding involuntarily are induced through hynotherapy.

www.cma.asn.au/glossary.htm

Meditation

This is the art of keeping the mind still and free of heavy thoughts. So many of us are preoccupied with thoughts of the past, future and present, exercising the mind too much. Imagine, the way we think is like doing a decathlon all day, every day. Our mind needs a break, like any motor. Energy drains from the brain and the consciousness we need to have to maintain a sense of peace.

Meditators exercise their ability to concentrate on only one thing, allowing the mind, body and spirit to synchronize in one place and rest at the same time. The effect can give an overall calmness, peace and sense of security that only comes when a person is connected at their very core. Without being religious, it can be very spiritual.

It has different forms. Using mantras - a spoken or sung phrase or tone - is very popular. The various tones a person uses align different parts of the mind, body and spirit.

Naturopathy

Naturopathy is a system of healing, originating from Europe, that views disease as a manifestation of alterations in the processes by which the body naturally heals itself. It emphasizes health restoration as well as disease treatment. The term "naturopathy" literally translates as "nature disease." Today naturopathy, or naturopathic medicine, is practiced throughout Europe, Australia, New Zealand, Canada, and the United States. There are six principles that form the basis of naturopathic practice in North America (not all are unique to naturopathy): www.naturesbridge.com/glossary.html

Naturopathy is a system, which is concerned with the whole person, rather than the problems afflicting his/her various organs and systems. Naturopathy recognizes and uses the fact that the body is a self-healing organism, working with the knowledge that if the right environment and opportunity for self-healing can be created; repair, recovery and good health will result.

www.footnotesforhealth.com/definitions.html

The Naturopath will have many different treatments to offer but all are based on the concept that the body will heal itself if given the right stimulus. A holistic system of healing that includes herbs, vitamins, massage, counseling as well as diet and nutrition. Naturopaths often give you an Iridological Diagnosis as part of the first consultation. Patients are treated as a whole person rather than just their symptoms.

www.institutenaturaltherapies.com/cmg.html

Organizing

You've heard the phrase "a place for everything and everything in it's place." For most of us, the phrase exists as an almost unachievable ideal.

If you've ever said "Someday I'm going to get organized," you need a professional organizer.

Professional organizers look at the way you already live your busy life then they help you configure your stuff (your files , your piles, your projects, possessions, papers, etc.) So that it works for you efficiently.

Professional organizers help create the structures that support you living your life efficiently and effectively. I believe that the quality of your physical environment and lifestyle reflects the level of health that you are able to enjoy. Look at your life, your car, your office, and your home; If you can say "My life is in order and organized," then you are likely to be very healthy. If you can not say that, get on the phone and find a professional organizer near you ASAP.

To find out more about professional organizing or to find an organizer in your area, see the website for the National Association of Professional Organizers (NAPO) www.napo.net or call (847) 375-4746.

Oriental Medicine

This science is well researched and has tremendous depth and breadth. There are many facets to it. In general, it is the management of the expression of "Chi", vital-life-sustaining energy thru 14 different medians and over 3,000 points on the body. It is a way of life, but treats specific conditions very effectively regardless of your lifestyle.

Personal Development Seminars

This trend is sweeping the planet. It is the future of Adult Education. There are workshops and seminars for anything you could imagine. Participating in workshops or seminars expands your intellectual and psychological vitality. Some expand the other aspects of vitality and viability.

There is a saying that people never change. [But] as more people are seeking to improve their lives by improving themselves, we are beginning to believe we can change. We are realizing we don't have to accept our "lot in life." We can do something about more consistently producing what we want in our lives.

Most of the organizations and individuals leading these seminars are legitimate and professional. These trainings and seminars should never be misconstrued as another religion or cult. They range in ideas from how to be a better professional to updating your belief systems. It's all about improving the quality of your life in some way. There are hundreds of professional companies, colleges and individuals giving seminars and workshops.

Psychotherapy

"A treatment by psychological means, of problems of an emotional nature in which a trained person establishes a professional relationship with the patient with the object of (1) removing, modifying, or retarding existing symptoms, (2) mediating disturbed patterns of behavior, and (3) promoting positive personality growth and development." (Wolber, The Technique of Psychotherapy, 1977

www.footnotesforhealth.com/definitions.html

Body-Oriented Psychotherapy seeks to enhance the psychotherapeutic process by incorporating a range of massage, bodywork and movement techniques. Acknowledging the mind/body link, practitioners may use light touch, softer deep-tissue manipulation, breathing techniques, movement, exercise or body-awareness techniques to help address emotional issues.

www.ticcenter.com/glossary.ivnu

Rebirthing (Breathwork)

Rebirthing-Breathwork, also called "Conscious Breathing", is a branch of alternative medicine which postulates that specialized breathing techniques may have theraputic benefits. In Rebirthing-Breathwork, the client makes a connected breath without a pause between inhale and exhale or between the exhale and inhale. According to practitioners, this causes a build up of prana or life energy. A state of deep peace & relaxation is achieved fairly easily by most. Breathing sessions are done lying down and usually last one to two hours.

It grew from the work of Leonard Orr. It was so named because when he first started doing this kind of work he noticed that he would often have what he describes as memories of his birth. Orr developed his process between 1962 and 1974 as he (without any (then) awareness of yoga or breathwork disciplines) discovered that modifications to breathing practices could bring about improvements in health, mental clarity and emotional well-being.

Development of Rebirthing as a therapeutic modality in its own right peaked in 1974, and has been extended from that point since. Orr, accompanied by fellow researchers, refined it into a system that can be practised in the context of a professional therapy session and taught to clients over a series of sessions, ten being the recommended minimum.

Proponents estimate that, since 1974, more than ten million people worldwide have learned the process, with more than one hundred thousand people completing practitioner training.

Two of the most popular evolutions of this breathwork are Clarity Breathwork and Holotropic Breathwork. For more complete definitions abd distinctions see www.breathwork.com or www.clarity.org

http://en.wikipedia.org/wiki/Rebirthing-Breathwork

Tantra

Tantra is the art of spiritual union through the sexual bond. It brings the sacredness to intimacy that makes romance satisfying and the sexual act fulfilling for each partner.

Through a series of processes and exercises, Tantra partners expand their awareness of their own sexuality and learn techniques that make sexual intimacy a mutually rewarding process.

For some it becomes the healing of personal wounds inflicted by early life experiences, society, religion or tradition. For others, Tantra is a doorway into a new world of experience that deepens, broadens, and intensifies romance and love.

For more information contact: Charles Muir
Source Tantra Seminars
Maui, HA
(808) 243-9851

12 Step Programs

The goal is to help people get control over their addictions and restore dominion over their lives. These programs are successful because they do several things in the same package. The sponsored person feels cared about. They acknowledge the existence of a higher power in a person's life. They encourage and cause a person to look within and access answers within themselves. They encourage the person to take full responsibility for the quality of life they create for themselves without mind-altering substances or practices. With all negative criticisms aside, the greatest value - no matter what the addiction - is in the community of caring that it raises and the self-reliance it fosters.

Yoga

This is a system of exercise and breath work which sometimes includes meditation. The goal is to open channels of energy that flow throughout the body. Technically, yoga is a very good way to enhance flexibility, balance and coordination in an organized way. It is a system of exercise. It focuses a lot on spiritual levels to synchronize the mind, body and spirit.

These few explanations are provided to be a quick, handy guide for any lay-person to use in getting started on the quest for life-enhancing services and skills to acquire. Create your own Personal Reference list as you get healthier and more vital with every new experience.

19

HOPE FOR THE FUTURE: The Completely Vital Consumer

There are products that come and go every year. I've seen them. You've seen them. I don't know how it is for you, but when I see these people coming with the same old song and dance about the amazing new product of the year, that they're really excited about sharing with you, I just yawn. Often enough, the company goes bust, my distributor vaporizes or the product doesn't do a thing for me.

Preface: There are hunderds, if not thousands of companies whose products could have easily been mentioned in this chapter. Go to my web site www.LivingWithVitality.com to read current product reviews and learn more about new developments and research being done by leading edge pioneers.

These days, I look for five key things when I choose products. I'll certainly try just about anything once, but I only tell my friends about the companies with products that have these vital ingredients:

Vision You Can Count on and Live By

Bodywise

The people at Bodywise remind me of the guy in Southern California who built a fireproof concrete house in a wooded house neighborhood in Malibu, California. The neighbors pointed and chuckled when he built the house many years ago. [But] after the great Malibu fire of 1995 burned and destroyed every home in the area for miles - except for his home - nobody laughed anymore.

The people at Bodywise specialize in products for people who expect to live a great life with health and quality for a long time. No glitz. No flaming hoops and cartwheels. No music. Just excellent products you can count on to help you reach your health and wholeness goals.

Integrity and Innovation

I believe that the quality of a company and its products will be reflected throughout the R&D, marketing, sales, service, supply-chain and the end users. The higher nature of the founders and developers will naturally attract the kind of distributors you would have as friends and invite into your home again and again.

There is a phrase in the New Testament of the Bible that reads: "By their fruits ye shall know them..." There are two companies that stand out in my mind, whose distributors were so impressive that I almost did not care what the product was. I just wanted to be affiliated with *them*, because their character spoke volumes about their intelligence, honesty, authenticity and effectiveness. Their company's product was an extension of a commitment to innovation and quality of life for everyone who comes in contact with their product.

Arbonne International

The idea to provide skin care products unparalleled in quality and effectiveness developed in Switzerland in 1975, when one man, Petter Mørck, together with a group of leading bio-chemists, biologists and herbalists, fulfilled his vision and founded Arbonne International. The proprietary formulas are owned by Arbonne and represent botanically-based products based on cutting-edge technologies and the latest advances in skin care science.

Arbonne makes Anti-Aging skin and body care products as well as aromatherapy, color, weight loss, and nutritional supplements. Arbonne's products are formulated in Switzerland, manufactured in California. The company currently has independent consultants in the United States, Canada and Puerto Rico. The unique thing about the entire product line is, the scientists asked: "What is the body trying to do for itself, to heal and regenerate the skin, hair and body tissues? Then they created products, drawing from the wealth of indigenous knowledge of botanical science, coupled with leading-edge scientific expertise and quality-control standards.

When you consider it, you might think, "Why doesn't everyone do it this way? I refer back to the commitment in the core values of the founders: Innovation and quality of life for everyone who comes in contact with their product. That is something I want in my life.

Nikken International

A dramatic event occurred in the life of Mr. Isamu Masuda during 1972. With the birth of his first child, this peaceful man grew concerned about health — his own (Mr. Masuda had been sickly as a boy), and the health of his family. Working as a clerk in the public transportation industry, he had to stretch a meager income. All this prompted him to look for a solution. He found it in a public bathhouse that had pebbles on the floor to create a natural massage effect on the feet. An idea was born.

In cooperation with Japanese scientists who had been studying magnetism, Mr. Masuda developed the prototype for a shoe insert, incorporating the pebble effect with magnets. As a pioneer in the evolution of this new system and with one unique product, Nikken came into being in Fukuoka, Japan, during March of 1975.

Recognizing the importance of peace, joy, *and* prosperity, Mr. Masuda synthesized his philosophy of balance in what he called the "5 Pillars of Health", which is at the core of the company mission. As a side-note: There is no exact translation from Japanese into the word "vitality", or even "wellness". Even so, I believe Mr. Masuda's core values will serve as a light that will guide humanity to complete vitality and quality lifestyle on many levels.

His 5 Pillars of Health are: Healthy Mind, Healthy Body, Healthy Family, Healthy Society and Healthy Finances. Instead of curing disease, total wellness focuses on prevention. It emphasizes not only better physical health, but peace of mind and financial security. According to Mr. Masuda, the key elements of physical vitality and the prevention of illness are: regenerative sleep, life-giving environment, proper nutrition and regular exercise. The objective is to keep these four areas in balance. When all are in harmony, the result can be a dramatic improvement in the quality of life. The company stretches the concept one step further by fostering the idea of the "Wellness Home". Offering a selection of wellness technology products, Nikken products provide an intelligent and practical approach to the challenges of modern living.

Resourcefulness and Simplicity

Cell Tech

Hmmmmm. A cold-water lake in Oregon that has an abundant source of unusual algae. What makes that stuff so special? What else can it do? What do they have? Where do they get it? Does it work? Does it taste good? How much of it do they have? Is it an unlimited and renewable source? What if I start using it regularly - how do I know they will be there as the demand for their product grows?

While I ask these kinds of questions of almost every product I try, I definitely went down my long list when I tried Cell Tech Super Blue Green Algae. The product's main ingredient is an algae that is a complete food by itself.

I'm impressed by the many products that have evolved from the use of this algae. What's even more significant is the continued research and the unsolicited testimonies I hear about from people who have used the various products in their time.

My Bottom Line

There are all kinds of products that hit the market every day. Yes, they make astounding claims sometimes. I've figured out for me that the only way to separate the cream from the crap, is to actually try stuff out.

I personally like to try new products after doing a little research on the internet, plus talking with a few people who tried the products. I believe every good product has a chance to suceed; and the useless products will usually go away quietly. Use your own rules, and try something new sometime soon.

For more information about these companies and distributors I know personally, see: www.LivingWithVitality.com

20

EPILOGUE: I Am A Novice At This.

The journey of a thousand miles begins with the first step. Whoever said that forgot to add the part about the detours, dead ends and pitfalls. There would be no map or compass on my trip—only angels. They seemed to appear just when I needed them most. I suspect they were there all the time.

Often I didn't know what to do or where to go next. I'd hear the voice of a friend saying, "Keep looking for the miracles." I'd reach out, and a hand would be there to support me to the next plateau, out of a tight spot or lead me to the place where my answers would be.

For whatever it's worth, "Keep looking for the miracles." Then hope, faith and action will let the angels know where to find you. [But] you must be committed to your complete vitality.

The quest for Complete Vitality is fun, exhilarating, rewarding and fulfilling. It is challenging, frustrating and a lot of work. I started out with the goal of knowing everything.

Now I feel like I've just started.

The most important thing I've learned on this voyage is this one secret:

Living with vitality is the destination of the thousand mile journey.

I'll be looking for you on the trail.— *Aaron*

About the Author

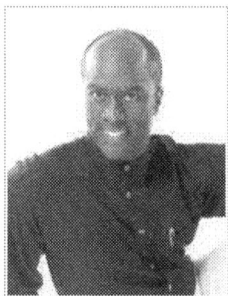

Aaron Parnell is one of today's emerging talents in the Vitality and Healthy Aging movement. *"The Vitality Man,"* is a dynamic and eloquent mind & body genius who captivates audiences, and gives clarity when you want vitality and pain-free living. Author of nearly 100 published articles, he has appeared on radio and TV across the nation. Aaron is one of 35 therapists chosen out of 2000 nationwide applicants for the first Olympic Sportsmassage team in Los Angeles. With over 20 years experience, Aaron is on a mission to help humanity thrive with vitality, fulfillment and longevity.

Performing some 300 interviews during the Olympiad, Parnell researched the thoughts, attitudes and actions of world-class athletes. This first-hand knowledge inspired Parnell to commit his career to helping everyone achieve extraordinary health. His ingenuity led him to develop innovative concepts such as *Reposturing Dynamics, ParaDyme Shift, Life Purpose/Life Work,* and more.

With a success-rate of nearly 100%, Parnell helps individuals improve their posture, sports performance and eliminate chronic pain *forever.* Through his Vitality Sciences Institute, he trains consumers in living the extraordinary health lifestyle, and certifies health professionals in providing services to consumers who want vitality.

As a vitality coach and fitness counselor, he assists clients in making lifestyle and work-style choices that lead to fulfillment and vitality.

A naturally gifted expert in ergonomics and body mechanics, Parnell helps companies save money and maximize workplace productivity.

In lectures, seminars and workshops "The Vitality Man" **educates and inspires consumers and health professionals** who want to help reverse the aging process, optimize sports-performance and gain freedom from pain.

Aaron Lloyd U. Parnell--*"The Vitality Man"*
CEO, Phyziquest Vitality Enterprizes, Inc.
407 North San Mateo Drive, San Mateo, California 94401-2417
Direct **(650) 347- 4565**
E-mail:**Aaron@LivingWithVitality.com**
Web site: **www.LivingWithVitality.com**